THE PLIABILITY STRETCH METHOD®

Mara Kimowitz

MENTOR
BUSINESS BOOKS

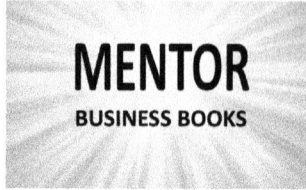

Manhanset House
Shelter Island Hts., New York 11965-0342

bricktower@aol.com • absolutelyamazingebooks.com

Library of Congress Cataloging-in-Publication Data
Kimowitz, Mara
The Pliability Stretch Method®
p. cm.

1. HEALTH & FITNESS / Exercise / Pilates.
2. HEALTH & FITNESS / Yoga.
3. HEALTH & FITNESS / Healthy Living. Non-Fiction, I. Title.

ISBN: 978-1-949504-44-6, Trade Paper

The Pliability Stretch Method® © 2025 by Mara Kimowitz

November 2025

Disclaimer

The techniques and methods outlined in this book, *Pliability Stretch Method®*, are intended for educational purposes only and should not be considered a substitute for medical advice, diagnosis, or treatment. Before beginning any new exercise or stretching program, consult with your physician or a qualified healthcare provider, especially if you have pre-existing health conditions, injuries, or concerns.

Stretching should always be performed mindfully and should never cause pain or significant discomfort. If you experience pain or any uncomfortable sensations while stretching, stop immediately and refrain from continuing until you have consulted with a medical professional. Your safety and well-being are paramount, and any concerns or symptoms should be promptly addressed by a licensed healthcare provider.

The author and publisher of this book are not responsible for any injury or harm that may result from the use or misuse of the information contained within. By engaging in the techniques described, you acknowledge and accept the risks involved and agree to take full responsibility for your own health and safety.

Stay safe, listen to your body, and enjoy the benefits of mindful stretching.

Endorsements

"Sadly, our modern society has become more and more sedentary, creating poor posture, altered musculoskeletal alignment and soft tissue restriction. We need to move our bodies to have optimal function and longevity, however, not all movement is created equal. The Stretch Lady, Mara Kimowitz clearly explains the value of assisted stretching through the Pliability Stretch Method® and why it is so beneficial for everyone to prevent injuries, stay active and heal from deconditioning or trauma. If you are interested in living a full, vibrant long life, you would benefit from learning more about this specific method of assisted stretching and how it can keep you healthy and strong.

Dr. Laura T Brayton, DC, CACCP, CSP, CSCP

"As an exercise expert with over 20 years of experience, I highly endorse the Pliability Stretch Method® for partnered stretching. The book "Pliability Stretch Method®" offers an impressive and valuable passive partner stretching technique that is both effective and innovative. I can attest to the profound benefits of their methods, which I liken to receiving a moving massage. It's a valuable resource for anyone looking to enhance their stretching routine with a partner."

Lois Manzella Marchitto, owner Fitness Knocking®

"Mara Kimowitz's knowledge of all things stretching is exceptional. Her methods are explained well, making it easy for the reader to apply the information to their clientele immediately. *The Pliability Stretch Method*® an essential resource for any bodywork practitioner who wants to provide assisted stretching safely and effectively." –

Dr. Susannah Pitman, DAc, Lac

"Exercise is the best medicine and stretching is the secret ingredient. Mara's techniques can help alleviate many painful conditions and lead to a healthier lifestyle."

- Dr. Michael Gutkin, MD Board Certified in Sports Medicine and Physical Medicine and Rehabilitation.

Dedication

To my DNA. Just as stretching expands our limits and wellness nurtures our whole selves, may you grow and flourish with every step you take. May you embrace the journey of life with flexibility and resilience and find balance and joy in every moment. This book is dedicated to you, my greatest inspirations.

Acknowledgments

I want to thank Alvin Ailey American Dance Center and School of American Ballet for giving me the education as a child that ignited my love for dance and healthy movement. Thank you to Bradley and Monson Physical Therapy for providing me an opportunity to learn rehabilitation techniques among the world's finest physical therapy providers and doctors. I also greatly appreciate the StretchSource community who inspire me to share my love for stretching.

Thank you to my book coach, Barry Cohen for keeping me on track with my book when life constantly attempted to derail me and my husband, Adam, for always being my number one support.

Foreword

When I was just three years old, my mother took me to a summer stage performance in our local town. The show was a ballet being performed by a professional dance company. That show opened my eyes to a world of movement, wellness, and well-being, igniting a passion that would shape the course of my life. By the age of 12, I had auditioned for and been accepted into the prestigious School of American Ballet. At 15, I earned a scholarship to the equally esteemed Alvin Ailey American Dance Theater. My journey continued with my first professional gig at 19 with the Mark Morris Dance Group.

During my time with the company, I had the privilege of accessing a range of bodywork providers, including physical therapists for injuries, chiropractors for adjustments before performances, massage therapists to alleviate tension, and stretch providers to keep our bodies limber and agile. This comprehensive approach to movement health was a revelation and became a cornerstone of my professional life.

However, upon retiring from dance, I found a gap in the resources available for maintaining healthy movement. While there were ample resources for physical therapy, chiropractors and massage therapists, there was a noticeable lack of resources for stretching. Yoga, though immensely valuable in its own right, primarily focuses on meditation, breathwork, and mental balance. While it incorporates stretching, its primary goal is not dedicated stretch training.

Driven by the need for a more focused approach, I embarked on a journey to create a resource specifically designed for stretching. I took on a job as a Physical Therapy Assistant at a prestigious NYC office to learn firsthand rehabilitation and movement techniques such as the Alexander and Feldenkrais Method. Over the course of a decade and through working with thousands of clients, I developed the Pliability Stretch Method®. This method is a comprehensive series of stretches tailored to meet the diverse needs of individuals across all body types, ages, and fitness levels.

In this book, I am excited to share not only the philosophy behind the Pliability Stretch Method® but also the demand for such a technique and the benefits it offers. My goal is to provide a valuable tool that enhances movement health and well-being, helping others achieve the same flexibility and balance that has been so transformative for me.

I hope this book serves as a guide and inspiration for those seeking to improve their flexibility and overall wellness through focused and effective assisted stretching or to providers looking to help people gain the same.

— Mara

Section 1

Chapter 1

The State of the Stretch Industry

1. The Emersion of Stretching

2. Common Assisted Stretch Methods

3. Assisted Stretching vs Other Methods

4. Summary

THE EMERSION OF STRETCHING

Assisted stretching is a 22-billion-dollar industry and growing. In just one year, close to 200 stretch franchises opened in the United States. Many of these companies have gone international. This proves that assisted stretching is not just a fad, but rather a real trend. It is here to stay and the public needs it.

Centuries ago, a person's ability to thrive was dependent on being active and outside the house. Farmers worked the land. People walked to their jobs or rode a horse. Now a days, you can have your food delivered with a click of a button, work from your home and even receive virtual medical care without stepping outside your door. Add on the pandemic of 2020 which found individuals spending more time watching TV, playing computer games, and generally sitting for longer periods of time. Individuals stopped exercising during the pandemic and became deconditioned. The modern-day sedentary lifestyle and pandemic have increased musculoskeletal issues and the need for focused stretching. A 2017 paper by the Sedentary Behavior Research Network (SBRN) defined sedentary behaviors as any activity involving sitting, reclining, or lying down that has very low energy expenditure. This type of low energy activity has impacted negatively peoples' sitting and standing posture. Excessive sitting is causing neck, hip, and low back issues. The prevalence of chronic low back pain more than doubled in a 14-year interval from 3.9 to 10.2 percent.
(https://www.ncbi.nlm.nih.gov/pmc/articles/PMC4339077/).

Pliability Stretch® Specialist are in a unique position to help people get over pain and injuries or gain the pliability necessary to resume exercise safely as a result of long periods of inactivity.

Stretching is not a new concept. Stretching has been around for centuries. However, years ago muscle issues were not a problem. It's only in modern times that people have become more sedentary. Stretching is no longer just a means to avoiding injury. It is used to reverse damage and dysfunction due to inactivity.

The Pliability Stretch® Method has helped thousands of people of all abilities, ages and fitness levels attain the pliability they need to participate in activities in life that make them happy without pain or limitation. Young athletes have a season injury free. Senior citizens can maintain independence and healthy aging with Pliability Stretch®. Even individuals with special needs such as cerebral palsy, spina bifida and wheelchair users benefit from the adaptability and customization of the Pliability Stretch Method®. It is the true method of assisted stretching for ALL.

Recent research shows that the method of Pliability Stretch® is associated with heart health. A 2009 study in the *American Journal of Physiology* showed that for people aged forty and over, flexibility in the body was accompanied by flexibility in the arteries, reducing the risk for cardiovascular disease and even death. Recent research from the University of Milan determined that passive stretching is shown to be an effective means to improve vascular function, with practical implications for its use as a novel non-pharmacological treatment for improving vascular health, reducing the overall cardiovascular risk, especially in individuals with limited mobility. Passive stretching refers to the use of an "outside agent" to administer the stretch such as a Pliability Stretch® Specialist. "This new application of stretching is especially relevant in the current post-pandemic period of increased confinement to our homes, where the possibility of performing beneficial training to improve and prevent heart disease, stroke and other conditions is limited," said study author Emiliano Ce at the University of Milan. This research shows how Pliability Stretch® could serve as a new drug-free treatment for improving vascular health and reducing disease risk.

Though there is no scientific theory supporting the increase in stretch popularity, the experience of the author may offer some insight. Back in 1998, Mara Kimowitz was pursuing a career as a professional dancer. She worked in the fields of physical therapy and fitness to pay for dance classes. She would go on to dance with renowned dance companies such as the Mark Morris Dance Group and Metropolitan Opera as well as be featured in music videos and commercials.

When Kimowitz retired from dancing, she returned to work as a personal trainer. As a personal trainer, she would provide strength training and cardio training for her clients. But what was different about her training sessions is Kimowitz also stretched her clients. Eventually, her clients began booking 30-minute and 60-minute stretch sessions as add-ons to traditional strength and cardio training because they saw the benefits. Benefits included improved performance, better recovery from activities, injury prevention and over-all better well-being. Other trainers began referring clients to Kimowitz just for stretching as well. Eventually, stretching clients is all she did! Kimowitz became known as "The Stretch Lady" – a title she proudly dons to this day. Exclusively through assisted stretching, Kimowitz made a living, supported a family, and a spouse through medical school. She developed the Pliability Stretch® Method over ten years and trialed it on over 1,000 clients.

Fast forward to now, fitness and wellness professionals who are students of Kimowitz are setting up tables in gyms, spas, medical offices and opening independent stretch studios. The success of her students has become noticed resulting in large investors backing businesses and franchises dedicated to assisted stretching. Pliability Stretch® remains an independent education company dedicated to supporting professionals looking to break into the industry, join a movement of like-minded individuals, and help more people. Though many of the assisted stretch businesses are successful, the growth business model associated with the establishments and larger enterprises has been detrimental to the quality control of the services. Many practitioners at these establishments receive fewer than 5 hours of training simply for-profit driven benefit. This is not considered adequate time needed to learn how to properly assess and create an individual and customized stretch program. The stretch services at such an establishment are considered generic, limited, painful and lack customization and quality control. In addition, often these establishments generate revenue by implementing other recovery tools and methods to make up for the lack of practitioner stretching skills. Just like any form of exercise, if not executed correctly, stretching can cause more harm than good. Having a system of stretching as well as a solid foundation of core principles is needed to ensure safe and maximum benefit.

This book is important in establishing clear direction, approach, and techniques that professionals can use with confidence. During today's stretching phenomenon, Pliability Stretch® Specialists are leading the industry in professionalism, quality, and best results. Unlike other methods that are geared to athletes, Pliability Stretch® is for everyone. Youth athletes looking to have an injury free season, empty nesters needing the pliability to play golf and tennis, senior citizens wanting to maintain independence and even severely handicapped individuals such as wheelchair users, all seek out Pliability Stretch®. For full access to the benefits of the Pliability Stretch® Method one needs to seek out or partake in a professional training with the Pliability Stretch® Academy.

COMMON ASSISTED STRETCH METHODS

Let's dive into some of the different methods of assisted stretching to better understand why Pliability Stretch® is a leader in the industry and the true method for ALL people. Assisted stretching is also referred to as partnered stretching where a stretching is executed with the assistance of another person. Often the recipient of the stretch is passive when a partner conducts the stretch. This approach to stretching is meant to allow the recipient's body to be moved in ways that would not be attainable when stretching alone.

FOUR TYPES OF STRETCHING TECHNIQUES

Techniques of stretching are used in medicine, wellness, and fitness. These are different than methods which are systems of stretching that will be discussed further in this section. There are four common techniques of stretching:

- Static stretching
- Dynamic stretching
- Proprioceptive Neuromuscular Facilitation (PNF)
- Ballistic Stretching

STATIC STRETCHING

Static stretching is considered the most common stretching technique. Static stretching is executed by adding force to the targeted muscle group so that the muscle extends to its maximum point and holding the stretch for fifteen seconds or more. This technique of stretching is recommended for use after a workout and exercise. The two types of static stretching are active and passive. Active static stretching is when added force is applied by the individual to oneself. Passive static stretching is when added force is applied by an external source to increase intensity and is commonly used in many assisted stretch methods. Static stretching is more beneficial when the muscles are warm and therefore is not recommended when cold or before exercise.

DYNAMIC STRETCHING

Dynamic stretching, unlike static stretching, requires the use of continuous movement patterns that mimic the exercise or sport to be performed. Generally, the purpose of dynamic stretching is to improve flexibility for a given sport or activity. Therefore, dynamic stretching is recommended before exercise or in the morning.

PNF

PNF stands for Proprioceptive Neuromuscular Facilitation. This technique of stretching is often taught in advanced levels of assisted stretch training and involves "contract and release" or "hold and relax" movements when stretching. According to the International PNF Association, (https://www.ipnfa.org/?id=113) PNF stretching was developed by Dr. Herman Kabat in the 1940's as a method of rehabilitating stroke victims and refers to any of the several post-isometric-relaxation stretching techniques. These are when a muscle group is passively stretched and then contracted isometrically against resistance, whilst it is in a stretched position to improve range of motion.

BALLISTIC STRETCHING

This type of stretching is reserved for top conditioned athletes to prepare for performance and is not considered safe for the average person. It uses a repetitive bouncing movement to gain greater range of motion. Whereas static stretches are performed slowly and gradually, the ballistic method stretches muscles much farther and faster and should be reserved for top athletes and medical professionals.

MOST RECONIZED METHODS OF ASSISTED STRETCHING TODAY!

A method, as described in this book is a system of stretching with specific procedures and philosophy. Each method of assisted stretching varies in its use of the four techniques previously mentioned and ultimate goals. Explaining the techniques used in each method will help create comparisons and differences. We will then share the techniques and goals associated with Pliability Stretch® positioning it as the method most suitable for people of all fitness levels, ages and abilities rather than just athletes.

The most common assisted stretch methods today are:

- Traditional Medical Stretching
- Fascial Stretch Therapy
- Thai Massage
- Pliability Stretch®

TRADITIONAL MEDICAL STRETCHING

The use of stretching for muscular re-training is associated with rehabilitation. Physical therapists use a combination of all four stretching techniques mentioned earlier to help patients recover from surgery and injury in combination with strength training, manual work, and other rehabilitation tools. Though a physical therapist is a highly skilled medical professional, often a doctor, with high level education of four-eight years, the stretching is focused on rehabilitation and not prevention. The focus of the stretching is usually specific to a prescribed area and not a holistic full body approach. It is typically used following a trauma, such as an automobile accident or surgery. Traditional medical stretching is performed on a treatment table.

FASCIAL STRETCH THERAPY

Fascial stretch therapy is generic term for a philosophy of assisted stretching that focuses on the connective tissue called "fascia". Fascia work originates with massage therapy and physical therapy. It has most recently been associated with assisted stretching. Fascial Stretch Therapy involves straps that retrain certain parts of the body so that a practitioner can access what is referred by the method as "the nets". "The nets", as described by training institutions, are all the bodily systems that are connected to the fascia. Whereas massage therapists and medical professionals use manual work to access the fascia, Fascial Stretch Therapy providers presume to use assisted stretching. Techniques used by the fascial stretch therapy method include static and PNF stretching on a table using straps.

THAI MASSAGE

Thai massage is one of the oldest forms of stretching still used today. It is believed that Thai Massage was developed more than 2500 years ago by Jivaka Kumar Bhaccha. Many of the Thai massage stretches are based on yoga poses with static passive stretching administered to increase flexibility, spirituality, and calm. A Thai massage practitioner will utilize all parts of their body including feet to execute stretches. Thai massage is usually conducted on the floor and not on a table and therefore recipients should have a degree of fitness and ability to get up and down from the floor safely and without injury.

PLIABILITY STRETCH®

Pliability Stretch® considers that not everyone needs to be more flexible to live active and pain free lives. More so, people need to be pliable. Everyone seeks out the ability to participate in activities in life that make them happy without physical limitation or discomfort. People want to be able to do this for longevity and independence of a lifetime. Pliability Stretch® Specialists help people attain these goals by helping them attain necessary pliability of their muscles through customized assisted stretching. Techniques used in the Pliability Stretch® Method include static passive stretching, dynamic stretching and PNF.

Pliability Stretch® targets muscle work to lengthen and soften every muscle in the body as the muscle is stretched and relaxed. The Pliability Stretch® Method believes natural pliability of the body needs to be attained organically and therefore there is no use of straps or other stretch accessories. Pliability Stretch® is conducted on a table since it was developed to be the assisted stretch technique for all types of people and abilities and someone with minimal pliability cannot be expected to get up and down from a floor safely.

Pliability Stretch® is often described as a marriage between a massage and physical therapy. Like massage, Pliability Stretch® is meant to relax the muscles and nervous system. Like physical therapy, the method sets out to reeducate the body to work more efficiently. Like other methods of pliability training that are endorsed by major athletes like Tom Brady, the goal of the Pliability Stretch® Method is to train the brain-body connection, which sends messages to the muscles to stay long, soft, and primed. You can think of it as the ultimate preparation and recovery for activities in life.

During a session, the specialist applies gentle force to lengthen and soften a client's muscles while they stretch and relax. This promotes oxygen-rich blood flow and anti-inflammatory responses in the moment. Through repetition, the Pliability Stretch® method strengthens the brain-body connection that tells muscles to stay pliable. Compared to short and dense muscles, long and soft muscles are better able to absorb and transfer forces they encounter in sports and everyday life. This enables patients to train and perform everyday activities with less risk of injury and pain.

The Pliability Stretch® book illustrates a series of stretches conducted with a partner that will make muscles less tight, dense, stiff and injury prone. Just as giving yourself a massage is very different than getting a massage, stretching on your own as in yoga and Pilates is very different then relaxing on a table while someone else does the work to unlock the tension in your body and help calm your nervous system. A calm nervous system promotes health and well-being. The parasympathetic nervous system controls the body's ability to relax and is referred to as the "rest and digest" state. This system is responsible for the body's response when relaxing, resting, or feeding. It is known to undo the work of the sympathetic division after a stressful situation. Whereas the sympathetic nervous system activates the fight or flight response during a threat or perceived danger, the parasympathetic nervous system restores the body to a state of calm. Pliability Stretch® taps into the body's calming system through holistic and gentle stretching techniques including passive static stretching, dynamic stretching and PNF. This is a huge difference between Pliability Stretch® and other methods of assisted stretching that are aggressive, painful, and unnatural.

Pliability Stretch® is an opportunity for you to give your nervous system a break and let someone else do the work for you.

ASSISTED STRETCHING VERSES OTHER METHODS

Pilates and Yoga are methods of exercise and wellness that incorporate stretching but do not have the same benefits as assisted stretching. Imagine an individual training for a marathon. The individual sets out on a long-distance run for training day. He runs for 10 minutes straight and then decides to pause to eat a healthy salad for 5 minutes. He resumes to run for another 10 minutes and again stops to eat a healthy salad. Eating a salad is healthy so it is all good, right? Wrong! There is no way the runner is going to improve his distance if he keeps stopping to eat a salad even if it is healthy for him. Same holds true for stretching. You will not experience the full potential of pliability, mobility, and flexibility if you are interrupting the stretching with other methods of exercise and wellness.

PILATES

The Pilates Method Alliance describes Pilates (pronounced puh-lah-teez and not pie-lates) as a method of exercise and physical movement designed to stretch, strengthen, and balance the body. This method of exercise is conducted either on the floor with a mat or machines. Within the description alone, Pilates is not focused stretch training and therefore will not have the same benefits as assisted stretching. Pilates focuses on strengthening as well as stretching and balance. Pilates is a valuable resource for conditioning and core training. However, like the runner, a person needs to dedicate time to focused stretch training to see full benefits. This is not the full focus with Pilates.

YOGA

As described by Wikipedia, yoga is a group of physical, mental, and spiritual practices which originated in ancient India and aim to control the mind. Yoga origins can be traced back to northern India over 5,000 years ago. Yoga is amongst the six schools of philosophy in Hinduism and is a major part of Buddhism and meditation practices.

Yoga holds a very important place in the world of wellness and health. In addition, especially in the western world, many elements of stretching have been added to the original practices of meditation and breathing. However, like the runner, stopping from stretching every few minutes for breathing and meditation exercises is not focused stretch training and therefore will not have the same benefits as assisted stretching.

PLIABILITY STRETCH®

Pliability Stretch® is a system dedicated to stretching and only stretching. The holistic method does not utilize outside tools or devices. It is all hands-on work. An individual relaxes on a table while someone else does the work to unlock tension, reduce pain, and improve pliability of the muscles. The system is based on the scientific principles of flexibility, mobility and pliability and is accredited by National Academy of Sports Medicine, Athletic and Fitness Association of America, and The National Certification Board for Therapeutic Massage & Bodywork.

SUMMARY

Assisted stretching has exploded in the fitness and wellness space in the last 10 years and has proven it's here to stay. Big investors are buying into the concepts, spas and gyms are adding it to offerings and medical professionals are referring patients for it. With any growing concept the issue is quality control. Many of these large, assisted stretch concepts are losing control over the qualifications and skills of the practitioners. Many lack ability to properly assess an individual's needs and offer a truly customized stretch program. Pliability Stretch® is strongly branded with strong core principles and proprietary assessment. Our proprietary Flex IQ™ assessment evaluates an individual's flexibility, range of motion, muscle health and history to create a truly customized stretch program. Our 4 core principles, T.E.A.M. – Tranquility, Evenness, Alignment and Mobility have proven to guide our Pliability Stretch® program successfully like no other method available today. Our practitioners are highly trained and have clear guidance for success in helping others live healthier and more active lives. Absent a similar pre-assessment, you risk creating a program that not only may fail to properly address the individual's personal needs but may in fact result in injury.

"People need pliability to participate in activities in life without pain or limitation"

The public needs the professionalism and expertise of a Pliability Stretch® Specialist now more than ever. What people don't need is another stretch program focusing on flexibility or fascia work. Not every person needs the flexibility to be able to kick their foot to their noise. People need *pliability*. The pliability to participate in activities in life without pain or limitation. People don't need more fascia work through stretching. Massage therapists and other medical professionals spend years studying and mastering fascia work. The same level of care cannot be attained within a few days of learning a stretching technique.

Though there is not a lot of scientific data surrounding pliability through stretching we have seen the benefits repeatedly. And it's not just for athletes. Thanks to the customized approach and the Flex IQ™ assessment, people of all ages and abilities continue to benefit from Pliability Stretch®. Youth athletes have experienced a season injury free. Empty nesters enjoy getting back into playing tennis, golf, travel and enjoying their newfound freedom without pain. Senior citizens remain independent and attain healthy aging. And even those with special needs such as Parkinson's, cerebral palsy, paralysis, and neurological damage have reported improvement and better quality of life through Pliability Stretch®. We hope to inspire others to continue to be able to offer safe and effective assisted stretch services that meet the highest standard, do not discriminate and are available to all people, all ages and all abilities.

Section 1

Chapter 2
Pliability Explained

1. Introduction

2. Pliability verses Flexibility

3. Pliability and Fascia Release

4. Summary

References:

https://pubmed.ncbi.nlm.nih.gov/2229943/ - pliability verses flexibility
A study showing the positive benefits of static passive stretching:
https://www.ncbi.nlm.nih.gov/pmc/articles/PMC8619362/ - introduction

INTRODUCTION

Function-ability and healthy activity for all ages, fitness levels and abilities does not come from flexibility or fascia work. The ability to move through life without pain and with full mobility starts with healthy pliability. Pliability affects the muscles' ability to lengthen, remain soft, and stretch during physical performance, range of motion and physical injury in healthy active individuals. The onset of a sedentary lifestyle due to work, family, or surgery will leave a person with insufficient mobility and increased muscle tension. Even with the completion of physical therapy, a person may continue to experience compensation issues related to the original prognosis or due to lack of comprehensive care. Often physical therapy care is directly focused on a particular prognosis and area needing rehabilitation. The lack of full body pliability has the potential to lead to injury and other musculoskeletal issues. Pliability Stretch® program is ideal for individuals' post-physical therapy or during care as well as after a period of sedentary living.

Stretching to improve mobility, and not just to feel good or for meditation, is directly related to the functionality of the muscles. Pliability Stretch® is a clinical approach to flexibility and mobility training and is adaptable for all abilities and ages. Pliability is not just for athletes. It is for an individual looking to play leisurely golf, a senior citizen looking to remain independent, avoiding falls, as well as for special populations of individuals looking to improve or slow-down progression of medical conditions.

Spasticity is one of the most frequent and displaying clinical manifestations of people with stroke, cerebral palsy, Parkinson's and other movement disorders. Spasticity results in shortening and tightening of muscles. Passive stretching is widely used for individuals with spasticity and belief that health of the muscles improved and lengthened. Recent research (J Pers Med. 2021 Nov; 11(11): 1074. Published online 2021 Oct 24. doi: 10.3390/jpm11111074) shows that prolonged passive stretching provided through customized programing like Pliability Stretch® has shown to improve spasticity and related conditions. Reports also showed improvement with gait, the risk of fall and pain, as well as mechanical and neural properties. Other research out of the University of Miami's Department of Exercise and Sports Sciences (https://www.ncbi.nlm.nih.gov/pmc/articles/PMC2685233/) showed that assisted stretching improved functional performance in elderly persons and improved range of motion.

PLIABILITY VERSES FLEXIBILITY

Pliability Stretch® Academy is committed to creating the world's most elite stretch practitioners who are a community of healers that help people gain the pliability they need to live active lives without pain or limitation. All people, not just athletes and able-bodied people need pliability. Age-related declines in range of motion are associated with decreases in pliability and activities of daily living performance. The progression of the Pliability Stretch® Academy courses give specialists the skills and tools to work with all people from youth athletes to senior citizens, and even special needs individuals managing both cognitive, neurological and movement disorders.

There are methods of assisted stretching that push the joints into extreme ranges of motion and focus on increasing flexibility. This type of stretching is suitable for athletes and young people. This approach to assisted stretching may feel good in the moment, but it doesn't change the way your body handles daily activities or re-train the functionality of the muscles. The Pliability Stretch Method® focuses on retraining the muscles in order to gain the movement necessary to conduct activities pain and injury free.

To put it in perspective, think of it this way:
Flexibility – How Far You Can Bend
Pliability – How Long Before You Break

Flexibility is a muscle's ability to lengthen passively through a range of motion. Imagine pulling a rubber band apart. How far the band pulls apart is the flexibility of the runner band.

"Pliability Stretch® aims to train the muscles to stay soft and supple with movement and activity. "

25

Pliability relates to your muscles' ability to adapt to the demands of the activity. Pliability is what enables a person to perform a movement repeatedly over the long term without putting oneself at risk of injury. It is not dependent on range of motion. It depends on resilience and recovery. So, imagine the rubber band again. Pull it apart and release it repeatedly. If the rubber band remains soft and subtle then it won't break. But if it becomes tight and strained with repetition, it will break. Pliability Stretch® aims to train the muscles to stay soft and supple with movement and activity.

All people of all body types, ages and abilities need pliability. All people do not need more flexibility. A 90-year-old does not need to be able to reach one's foot to one's nose like the flexibility necessary for a gymnast or a dancer. However, all need pliability to perform and manage the demands of activities in life without pain or limitation. This is the importance of pliability verses flexibility.

PLAIBILITY AND FASCIA RELEASE

Fascia release work has been around a long time and in the past most associated with methods of massage and physical therapy. It is only in the last ten years that fascia work has been referenced in accordance with assisted stretching. Fascia attaches, encloses, and separates muscles and other internal organs, allowing these structures to slide and move through the body. When fascia is healthy, it's flexible enough to twist, glide and bend. One would consider any type of stretching, including yoga even, to provide some degree of fascia release.

Pliability Stretch® is therefore also a form of fascia stretch release. All types of stretching will help reduce the risk of inflammation and fascial issues. Pliability Stretch® technique benefits the flexibility of the fascia as well as the pliability of the muscles. It is both the fascia and the muscles that need to be healthy to fully gain the ability to participate in activities with healthy movement.

SUMMARY

Flexibility training and fascia work may seem synonymous with pliability, but they are not. Having the flexibility to reach your toes may be a cool trick, but not everyone needs that skill to live an active and healthy life. Fascia work may be good for breaking up fascia tension but will not change how the body manages movement. Pliability training is what your body needs to learn how to move without limitation or pain. Pliability Stretch® is the only method of assisted stretching that re-teaches the muscle how to work better and more efficiently. Other methods of assisted stretching such and Thai massage and fascia stretch focus only on flexibility and the fascia. These methods of assisted stretching do not take into consideration the re-training of the muscles like Pliability Stretch®.

Section 1

Chapter 3

Pliability Stretch Method®

1. Introduction

2. History

3. Four Core Principles – T.E.A.M.

4. Tranquility

5. Evenness

6. Alignment

7. Mobility

INTRODUCTION

In this chapter we explain the fundamental concepts and history of Pliability Stretch®. This includes the dissection and explanation of the four core principles and overall philosophy of the system. Once you understand the concepts and philosophy it will be easier to effectively execute and interpret the techniques in Section 2.

HISTORY

Pliability Stretch® creator, Mara Kimowitz, first conceptualized a stretching program in 1998. She was working alongside top industry Physical Therapists offering some of the best rehabilitation treatment available in New York City. Even with the top-notch care and having been compliant with execution and completion of treatment, many patients would return months later re-injured. In addition to rehabilitation, people needed preventative care. There was a gap in the fitness and medical industry and Kimowitz set out to fill it.

It would take a decade of research and two other careers for Kimowitz to develop a technique that would fill the gap. Using over twenty years of experience as a professional dancer, a Certified Personal Trainer, Group Fitness Instructor, Pilates Instructor, Pre-natal and Post-natal Fitness Specialist, and Triathlete Coach; Mara created Pliability Stretch®. Pliability Stretch® is in its own category of fitness and wellness. It is not flexibility training or Physical Therapy. It is the only training of its kind that focuses on pliability and improved functionality through assisted stretching.

Physical Therapists are the most trained professionals in stretch training and often attain a doctorate degree. Physical Therapy caters to the injured and those needing rehabilitation. Other forms of assisted stretching cater to sports performance and athletes. What about the rest of the population? What about the everyday empty nester looking to improve pliability in order to play tennis or golf? Or a senior citizen looking to maintain independence? Where do people go for the best stretch training outside of a PT prescription? Pliability Stretch® is the answer.

Pliability Stretch® ensures the safety, benefit, and consistency of its services through extensive training of providers. There is no other stretch method offering the same level of quality care and expertise.

By becoming a Pliability Stretch® Specialist you can be proud to be part of the best-of-the-best, a great network and team of professionals and increase the quality of life of your clients. Pliability Stretch® Workshops are offered so you can join the stretch movement and help more people. Pliability Stretch® was officially developed in 2017 by Mara Kimowitz. Fitness and wellness professionals can get certified in the method through the Pliability Stretch® course. The course begins with Level 1 and progresses to a Level 2 Corrective Exercise Specialist, and finally, a Level 3 Medical Specialist. Level 3 practitioners can help people of all abilities, including those managing severe medical conditions. Professionals receive continuing education credits thanks to an affiliation with several national organizations including the National Certification Board for Therapeutic Massage and Bodywork (NCBTMB), National Academy of Sports Medicine (NASM), Athletic and Fitness Association of American (AFAA), and (NCCAOM).

FOUR CORE PRINCIPLES – T.E.A.M.

There is no I in TEAM. As a Pliability Stretch® Specialist you are creating your own TEAMS within your profession. You have your professional team, which includes the Pliability Stretch® Network of professionals who are available to support and guide you. You also have your clients who become your teammates each time they see you. It is imperative to the safety of each client that you work as a team with open communication, respect and understanding.

Pliability Stretch® prides itself on four core principles that inspire our specialists to become leading professionals in this neglected category of fitness and wellness. Apply each of the principles to each of your clients and their progress is quite simply…guaranteed! Pliability

Stretch's® four core principles outline the criteria that guide all training and business.

Tranquility
Evenness
Alignment
Mobility

TRANQUILITY

Stretching should always feel good. Pliability Stretch® should feel like a wonderful massage. Creating calm in the body comes from deep and continual **BREATHING**. We are most relaxed when we are breathing fully and efficiently. Breathing should be natural and continues during stretching, never holding one's breath or tightening in the chest. If tension is exhibited in the body, then a stretch needs to be modified for comfort. Tranquility ensures calmness of the nervous system allowing the full benefits of stretching. Tranquility also refers to the ability of the muscles to remain soft during movements thus releasing tension. Additional ways to facilitate tranquility during a stretch session include playing relaxation music as well as aromatherapy.

EVENNESS

Pliability Stretch® is not flexibility training, it is stretch training. Flexibility training is about increasing flexibility, sometimes to extreme levels. A gymnast or dancer may need such training. Pliability Stretch® training is about creating a physiological balance and evenness based on the client's needs. Pliability Stretch® is not just for athletes. It is for everybody. Evenness, in nature, is never symmetrical since the human body is imperfect in nature. If a person is uneven, they will exhibit extreme difference in degrees of ROM (range of motions) from the left side to the right side or front to back.

We want to attain evenness at its best with the understanding that perfection is unrealistic.

ALIGNMENT

Stretching should not be conducted without good anatomical alignment and positioning. Constantly rechecking alignment is a significant part of executing stretches effectively. Proper alignment will be discussed further in Chapter 4.

MOBILITY

Pliability Stretch® philosophy of stretch training focuses on improvement of one's pliability and less so on one's flexibility. Flexibility refers to the ROM around a joint. Stretching often refers to actively attempting to increase ROM. There are a lot of conflicting expert opinions as to whether actively attempting to increase ROM around a joint is safe or necessary. Opinions vary depending on how an individual's ROM compares with normal ROM for the same joint. It depends on over-use or under-use of specific muscle groups due to a person's lifestyle. It depends on injuries. It depends on an individual's goals.

Stretching for mobility is about providing the pliability an individual needs to attain the most functional and healthy physical ability possible. **We stretch for mobility, function ability, pliability, and ultimately optimal performance.**

Mobility, for us, refers to the total range of motion through which a particular joint moves and is evaluated during a Flex IQ® Session.

Pliability Stretch® priority is not creating extreme or unnecessary flexibility for clients. It's about creating pain-free and functional mobility based on the individual's pliability needs. Each client will have unique pliability needs depending on profession, personal lifestyle and or fitness goals. Previous injuries will also play a role in a client's needs and customized stretch.

Section 1

Chapter 4

Muscle Physiology

1. Basic Anatomy

2. How Physiology Affects Stretching

3. Stretch Techniques

BASIC ANATOMY

Human movement is dependent on the amount of ROM available in joints. Range of motion, in general, is limited by two anatomical entities: joints and muscles. There are many reasons for decreased ROM, which we will discuss in greater length in the Level 1 Pliability Stretch® Course.

One of the many plausible causes of limited ROM is muscular tightness. Muscle provides both passive and active tension. Muscle "tightness" results from an increase in tension or passive mechanism, which may cause muscles imbalances. Muscle imbalances and dysfunction cause poor performance and a higher risk of injury.

Attaining pliability of the muscles helps improve the ROM of the joints and eliminate pain.

Muscle Anatomy
The human body contains over 215 pairs of skeletal muscles. Skeletal muscles can be broadly classified into two types: stabilizers and mobilizers.

Stabilizer- essentially stabilizes a joint and includes multifidus, transverses abdominals, gluteus maximus and adductor magnus.

Mobilizers- responsible for movement and includes the hamstrings, piriformis, and rhomboids.

Muscle Movements that yield action:
1. Concentric Contraction
2. Eccentric Contraction
3. Isotonic Contraction (Holding in concentric position)
4. Isometric Contraction (Holding in eccentric position)

Most important is that muscles need to be in full resting position with **NO CONTRACTION** to get the most benefit from the stretch. This is the main benefit of assisted stretching versus stretching yourself.

Stretching is basically improving muscle pliability by elongating the muscle fibers to maximum resting length, thus allowing connective tissue and muscle fascia to lengthen as well.

HOW DOES PHYSIOLOGY AFFECT STRETCHING?
When customizing a stretch program and treating a client it is important to consider all parts of the body and how they stack-up – literally! The Pliability Stretch® proprietary Flex IQ® stretch session is an assessment that provides valuable feedback to determine modifications or needs of the clients. Let us discuss some of the findings that may appear during a Flex IQ® stretch.

Postural Alignment:

A client's posture is going to be a big indicator of areas of tightness in the torso.

Postural alignment is the way in which one stands or sits. It can be affected by anatomical issues such as scoliosis and from poor body mechanics.

Kyphosis is an extreme rounding of the upper back that is usually accompanied by a forward head position. Tightness in the chest, neck, and lower back are often associated with kyphosis. Stretches that create better pliability of these muscles will help alleviate imbalances.

Lordosis is an extreme curve of the lower back that is often accompanied by weak abdominal muscles. Tightness in the buttocks, hamstrings, and hips are often associated with this position, therefore, stretches that create pliability of these muscles will help alleviate imbalances.

Alignment is never perfect. Good alignment means no apparent extremes of lordosis or kyphosis.

Pelvic Alignment:

As you observe a client's physiology, the next area of the body is the pelvic area. You want to check for extreme degrees of internal or external rotation in the hip joint. This is determined by checking the direction the client's knees point.

For example, if a person walks or stands with extreme external rotation, this is when the toes or knees face outwards, then inefficient internal rotation is present. A person uses internal rotation to walk, run, squat, crouch, and crawl. Inefficient internal rotation can lead to gait issues and injury. Stretches from the Pliability Stretch® technique can be used to improve the pliability and range of the muscles that rotate the hip inwards.

Foot Alignment:

Extreme pronation or supination of the feet should also be noted. Pronation or supination can also cause tightness in the lower back and hips as well as the ankle joint. One such Pliability Stretch® client was a 13-year-old field hockey player and complained of knee and back pain. She had been seen by every doctor and had every possible diagnostic test including x-rays. She had been seen for 63 physical therapy appointments over the course of 6 months without any improvement. Her parents were beginning to think the pain was in her head! Coming for Pliability Stretching® was her last chance for relief. During a Flex IQ® Stretch it was determined that her ankles were out of alignment because she had fallen arches of her feet. The fallen arches were causing muscles in her legs, hips and back to work extra hard and become rigid and tense. She received orthotics to support her feet and stretches that improved the pliability of the muscles that had been affected. Her pain went away!

STRETCH TECHNIQUES

Static Stretching - Considered the most common stretching technique; static stretching is executed by extending the targeted muscle group to its maximal point and holding it for 30 seconds or more.

There are two types of static stretches:

- **Active:** Added force is applied by the individual for greater intensity
- **Passive:** Added force is applied by an external force, for example a stretch provider, to increase intensity.

Dynamic stretching - Dynamic stretching, unlike static stretching, requires the use of continuous movement patterns that mimic the exercise or sport to be performed. Generally speaking, the purpose of dynamic stretching is to improve flexibility for a given sport or activity.

An example of dynamic stretching would be a sprinter doing long, exaggerated strides to prepare for a race.

PNF - Proprioceptive Neuromuscular Facilitation (**PNF**) is a more advanced form of flexibility training that involves both the **stretching** and contraction of the muscle group being targeted. **PNF stretching** was originally developed as a form of rehabilitation and for that purpose it is very effective.

Ballistic Stretching - This type of stretching is typically used for athletic drills and utilizes repeated bouncing movement to stretch the targeted muscle group. While these bouncing movements usually trigger the stretch reflex and may cause increased risk for injury, they can be safely performed if done from low-velocity to high-velocity and preceded by static stretching.

Section 2

Chapter 1

Flex IQ®

INTRODUCTION

The Pliability Stretch® Series is made of more than 30 stretches divided into 4-part series. The stretches and series can be altered and modified for customization and personalization. Therefore, an assessment is crucial to long tern retention. Personalization is the start and the only thing that will sustain your profession as a stretch provider. Pliability Stretch® Specialists are leaders in the industry because they have the unique ability to assess and customize stretching.

The Flex IQ® is a person's unique measurements of pliability, flexibility, and mobility. These measurements guide the creation of a customized stretch program. A Flex IQ® Assessment is the gathering of important information about goals, lifestyle habits, fitness level, and any limitations. This information will help you begin thinking about how you can help him or her. When you take the time to perform a Flex IQ® Assessment, you demonstrate value in your service and your ability to influence someone to invest in assisted stretching with you is greatly enhanced. That value will keep retention rates high. How to best sell stretching services is further discussed in the Pliability Stretch® Level 1 Course.

There are three parts to a comprehensive Flex IQ® Assessment. It takes approximately 60 minutes to complete and includes a verbal, practical and visual assessment. The three parts work together and provide you all the information you need to build a customized stretch program that will deliver results.

Setting up your workspace for success is an important part of providing quality services. Pliability Stretch® sessions are conducted on an oversized 40" firm treatment table. A client remains fully dressed and is recommended to wear grippy socks. The session can be conducted in a public space unless the client requests privacy. An open gym or shared space is acceptable. A towel for the client's head is recommended for hygiene and maintenance of the table surface. A full-body mirror is helpful in giving clients a visual understanding of proper body positioning.

The client's experience begins the moment he or she steps in the door. A clean and inviting space needs to be created. You should welcome the client as soon as he or she enters the facility. Show him or her where to place his or her items. Ask if he or she would like a bottle of water.

PART 1 – VERBAL ASSESSMENT

Basic health, wellness and fitness information should be collected, recorded, and discussed. This includes medical history, past injuries, present pain, and physical limitations. A person's fitness activity level and habits should be recorded as well as his or her goals. Level 1 students receive a copy of the Pliability Stretch® assessment forms.

When talking with your client make sure to ask as many questions as possible. The more details you have the better your ability to create a highly customized and valued stretch program. The information will help identify any contraindications to certain stretches.

Use the verbal assessment to explain Pliability Stretch®, the four core principles, and what the client can expect during the session.

PART 2 – PRACTICAL ASSESSMENT

Assessment of range of motion, muscle health and flexibility are crucial in creating attainable goals. The practical assessment includes measurements of the entire body including upper and lower joints.

These measurements are recorded and used to further customize a stretch program.

HAMSTRING EVALUATION

Goal: Measure the range of motion of the hip and pliability of the hamstring based on when the client begins to feel a stretch.

Client position: Supine with straight legs

Practitioners:
1. Raise the client's straight leg off the table.
2. Continue to raise the leg until a client begins to feel a stretch.
3. Make sure the client remains relaxed and does not help you as you lift the leg into a stretch.
4. Record the degrees of angle the leg height reached of the leg away from the table.
5. Make sure the client remains relaxed and does not help as you lower the leg back to starting position.
6. Repeat other side.

Observations: A client feels tension in the front of the hip during the hamstring evaluation may be an indication of tight psoas. A client who feels tension in the back of the hip/ buttocks/ back is an indication of a possible tight piriformis muscle.

Health of muscle: The goal of a healthy hamstring for a healthy active individual is 90 degrees from the table.

IT BAND EVALUATION
Goal: Measure the range of motion of the hip and pliability of the ITBAND based on when the client begins to feel a stretch in the IT Band.

Client position: Supine with straight legs

Practitioners:
7. Raise the client's straight leg to a comfortable 30% angle and then move across the body.
8. Continue to move leg across the body until a client begins to feel a stretch.

9. Make sure the client remains relaxed and does not help you as you lift the leg into a stretch.
10. Record the degrees of angle the leg height reached away from midline.
11. Make sure the client remains relaxed and does not help as you lower the leg back to starting position.
12. Repeat other side.

Observations: A client who feels tension in the back of the knee indicates tension in the knee joint. A client who feels tension in the lower back indicates possible tight piriformis muscle. Tension felt in the hamstring means leg might need to be lowered during stretch. Tension felt in the groin means leg might need to be raised higher during stretch.

Health of muscle: The goal of a healthy IT Band for a healthy active individual is 90 degrees from the medial line.

QUADRICEP EVALUATION
Goal: Measure the range of motion of the hip and pliability of the quadricep based on when the client begins to feel a stretch in the quadricep.

Client position: Prone with straight legs

Practitioners:
13. Raise the client's foot towards the buttocks as the knee bends.
14. Continue to bend the knee until the client begins to feel a stretch.
15. Make sure the client remains relaxed and does not help you as you lift the leg into a stretch.
16. Record the degree of angle of the bend.
17. Make sure the client remains relaxed and does not help as you lower the leg back to starting position.
18. Repeat on the other side

Observations: If a client's buttock tightens and there is movement observed in the back and hips then this indicates possible dysfunction of the psoas and piriformis muscles.

Health of muscle: The goal of a healthy quadricep for a healthy active individual is 180 degrees from starting position. This means the foot bends all the way to the buttocks.

CALF EVALUATION

Goal: Assess the pliability of the gastrocnemius based on the tension of the ankle joint.

Client position: Prone with straight legs

Practitioners:

19. Raise the client's foot into a comfortable bend of the knee.
20. Press gently on the foot to create a 90% flexion of the ankle joint.
21. Press further to observe pliability of the joint and ability to flex beyond 90%.
22. Record findings.
23. Repeat on the other side

Observations: If the ankle joint does not flex beyond 90% then there is dysfunction of the muscles.

Health of muscle: The goal of a healthy ankle joint is flexion beyond 90% without pain, limitation, or restriction.

POSTURE

Goal: Assess postural alignment

Client position: Standing against the wall, feet a few inches away from the wall, feet hip width apart, knees slightly bent and head against the wall. Elbows lifted in line with the shoulders and wrists in line with the shoulders.

Practitioners:
4. Observe if the chin is raised and neck stuck in flexion.
5. Observe if the back is against the wall or there is tension in the spine.
6. Observe any tension or pain in the shoulder or neck.
7. Observe any postural misalignment in the upper and lower body.
8. Record findings.

Observations: A chin stuck in neck flexion is an indication of lack of pliability in the cervical spine. Shoulders lifted off the wall is indication of lack of pliability of the pectoralis muscles. Raised shoulders is indication of tension in the trapezius muscles. Pain in the trapezius/neck indicates lack of pliability in the thoracic spine muscles. Lower back lifted off the wall is indicating tension in the lumbar spine and possible psoas tension.

Health of muscle: The goal of a healthy postural alignment is chin parallel to the floor, back against the wall, entire spine pressed against the wall, no tension in the neck, upper or lower back with standing position.

ROTATOR CUFF
Goal: Assess the health of the shoulder joint based on the pliability of the rotator cuff.

Client position: Standing against the wall, feet a few inches away from the wall, feet hip width apart, knees slightly bent and head against the wall. Elbows lifted in line with the shoulders and wrists in line with the shoulders.

Practitioners:

1. Ask client to rotate shoulders and bring hands towards the wall to make a goalie post position.
2. Observe how far the client can reach to the wall.
3. Observe any tension or pain in the shoulder or neck or imbalances.
4. Record findings.

Observations: Observe any imbalances of left and right. Observe any tension in the muscles. Pain in the upper spine indicates thoracic spine tension.

Health of muscle: The goal of a healthy rotator cuff and shoulder joint is the ability to touch the wall with a 90% elbow bend and rotation.

DELTOID

Goal: Assess the health of the shoulder joint and pliability of the deltoids.

Client position: Standing against the wall, feet a few inches away from the wall, feet hip width apart, knees slightly bent and head against the wall. Keep the hands reaching towards the wall in the rotator cuff assessment position.

Practitioners:

1. Ask the client to raise the hands up into a diamond position over head.
2. Observe any tension or pain in the shoulder or neck.
3. Observe any imbalances.
4. Record findings.

Observations: Observe if there is any indication of imbalances from right to left and any tension in the neck, back or shoulders.
Health of muscle: The goal of a healthy deltoids and shoulder range of motion is the ability to create a diamond over head with elbows and hands against the wall as well as the spine and head against the wall.

48

PART 3 – VISUAL ASSESSMENT
Healthy pliability is determined by the muscles' ability to remain soft and long during activity. The way the joints and muscles work together is very important in creating functional ability and quality of life. During the visual assessment a client is taught to execute a dynamic stretch warm-up. Modifications to the warm-up for clients with mobility restrictions is taught in the Level 1 Pliability Stretch® Specialist Course.

DYNAMIC STRETCH WARM-UP (See next chapter for further guidance)

1. Standing position
2. Double Thumbs Up Marching
3. Arm Circles Backwards and Forwards
4. Titanic Chest Stretch
5. Zipper Down
6. Forward Fold
7. Plank
8. Downward Dog
9. Child Pose
10. All Fours to Forward Fold
11. Zipper Up

Goal: Create warmth in the muscles to maximize benefits of assisted stretching. Client should only attempt movements that are comfortable and non-strenuous.

Client Movement: Please see next chapter for full explanation.

Practitioners:

1. See next chapter for full description of assisted stretches.
2. Observe and record movement quality, imbalances, tension, and any limitations.

Observations: A chin stuck in neck flexion is indication of lack of pliability in the cervical spine. Shoulders lifted off the wall is an indication of lack of pliability of the pectoralis muscles. Raised shoulders is an indication of tension in the trapezius muscles. Pain in the trapezius/neck indicates lack of pliability in the thoracic spine muscles. Lower back lifted off the wall is indicating tension in the lumbar spine and possible psoas tension.

Health of muscle: The goal of a healthy postural alignment is chin parallel to the floor, back against the wall, entire spine pressed against the wall, no tension in the neck, upper or lower back with standing position.

Section 2

Chapter 3

Dynamic Warm-up

1. Introduction
2. Double Thumbs Up Marching
3. Arm Circles
4. Titanic
5. Zipper Down into Forward Fold
6. Plank
7. Downward Dog
8. Child Pose
9. All Fours to Forward Fold
10. Zipper Up

INTRODUCTION

A person should never be stretched cold. A dynamic stretch warm-up is considered the most beneficial way to get the body ready for active stretching. The warm-up is introduced to a new client during the evaluation. The provider should continue to offer cues and guidance at each session. During each new session, the provider will use the warm-up as a re-assessment of a client's physical conditions and needs.

Beginning Position
The warm-up begins with the client standing hip width apart, feet parallel and a natural weight of arms by the side.

DOUBLE THUMBS UP MARCHING
Stretch Technique

- Cue proper arm movement - thumbs up, evenness, natural swing
- Cue proper march movement – opposite arm and leg, lift knee to comfortable height to feel stretch in opposite quad (Those with mobility limitations may hold onto a chair or wall)
- Freeze and balance every couple of odd number marches
- Resume each side

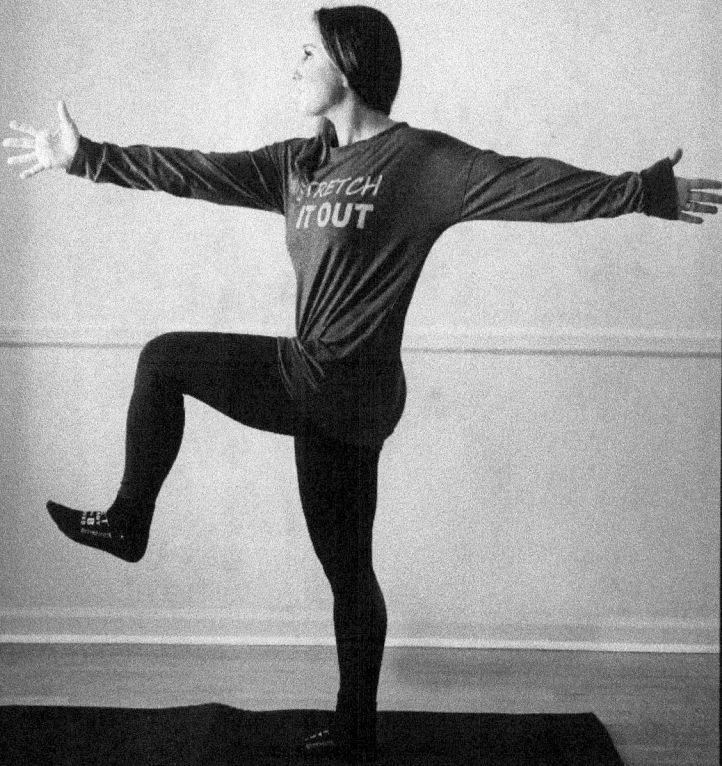

pliability stretch®

MARCHING

DOUBLE THUMBS UP

Assisted Stretch Technique
- Cue client to take a deep breath in
- Upon exhale hold the client's arms above the elbow and gently increase the stretch in opposition (ahead and behind)

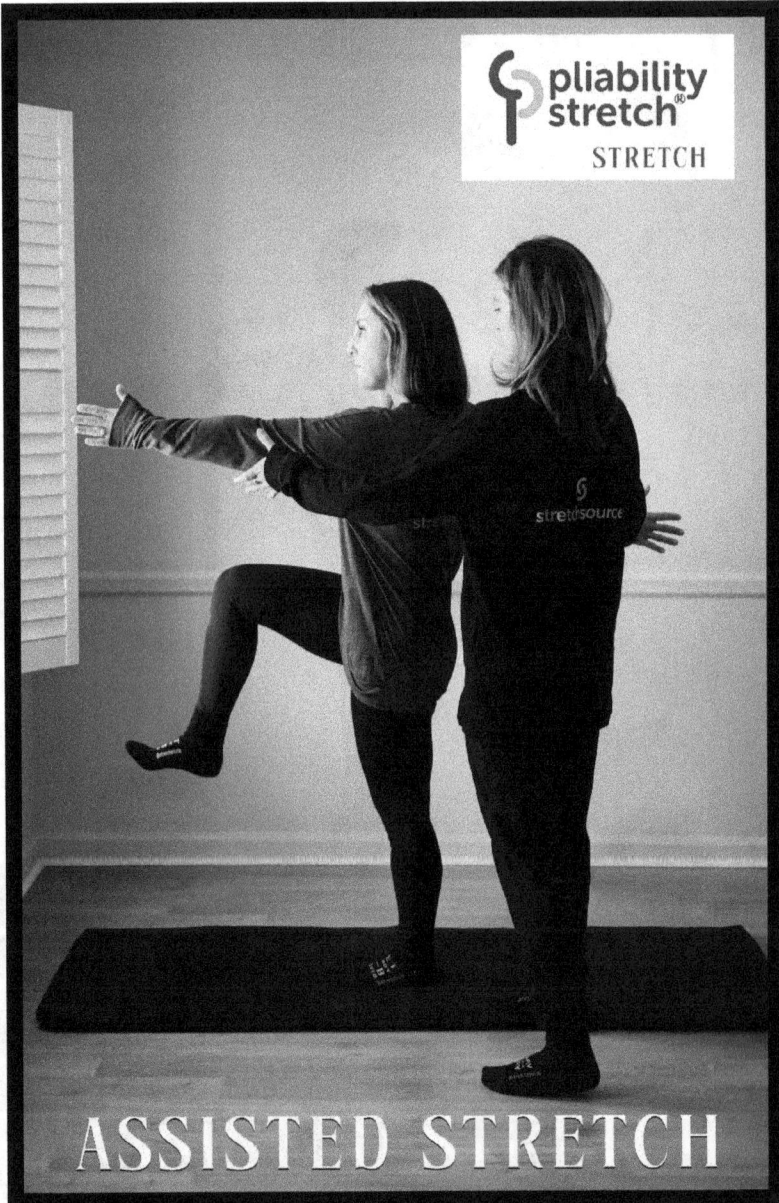

ASSISTED STRETCH

ARM CIRCLES
Stretch Technique
- Cue your client to stand parallel with knees slightly bent, and to circle arms in backward and to stop arms parallel forward shoulder height (Sitting for limited mobility)
- Cue your client to circle arms forward stroke and to stop with arms out to either side in line with the shoulders
- Repeat as needed

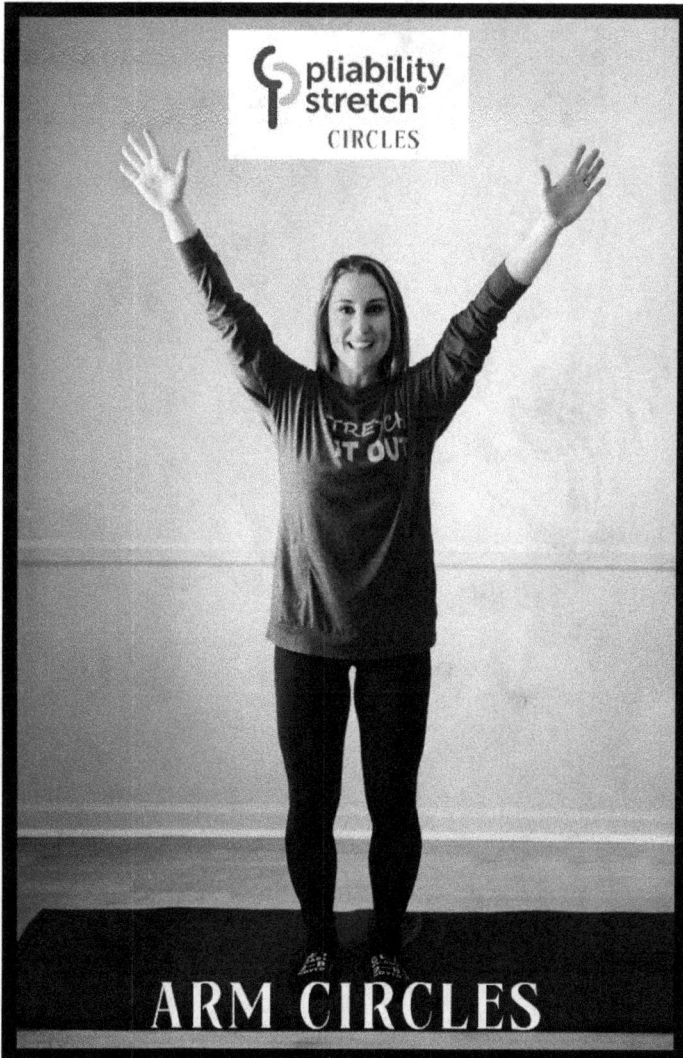

Assisted Stretch Technique
- Place your hands on the shoulders
- As the client executes backwards motion help facilitate the opening of the sternum, chest and shoulders

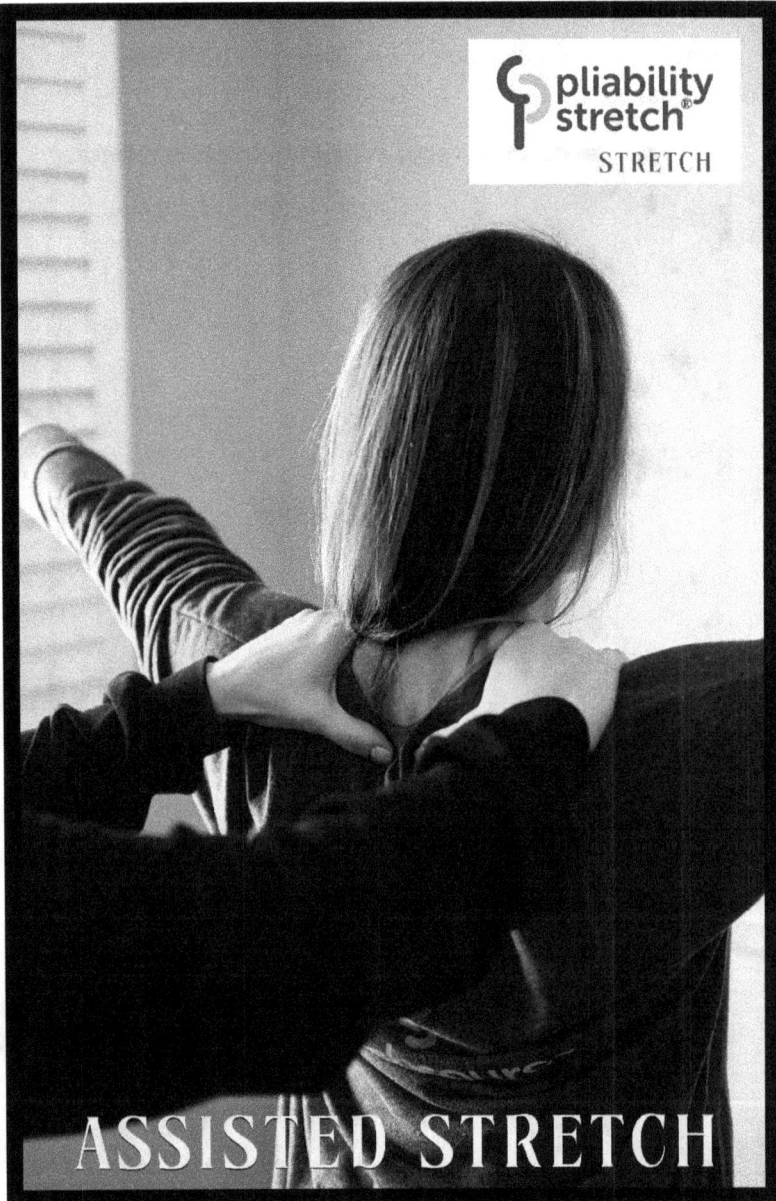

TITANIC
Stretch Technique
- Cue client to hold arms out in t-shape and life chest and chin.
- Add manual stretch to neck, spine and chest.

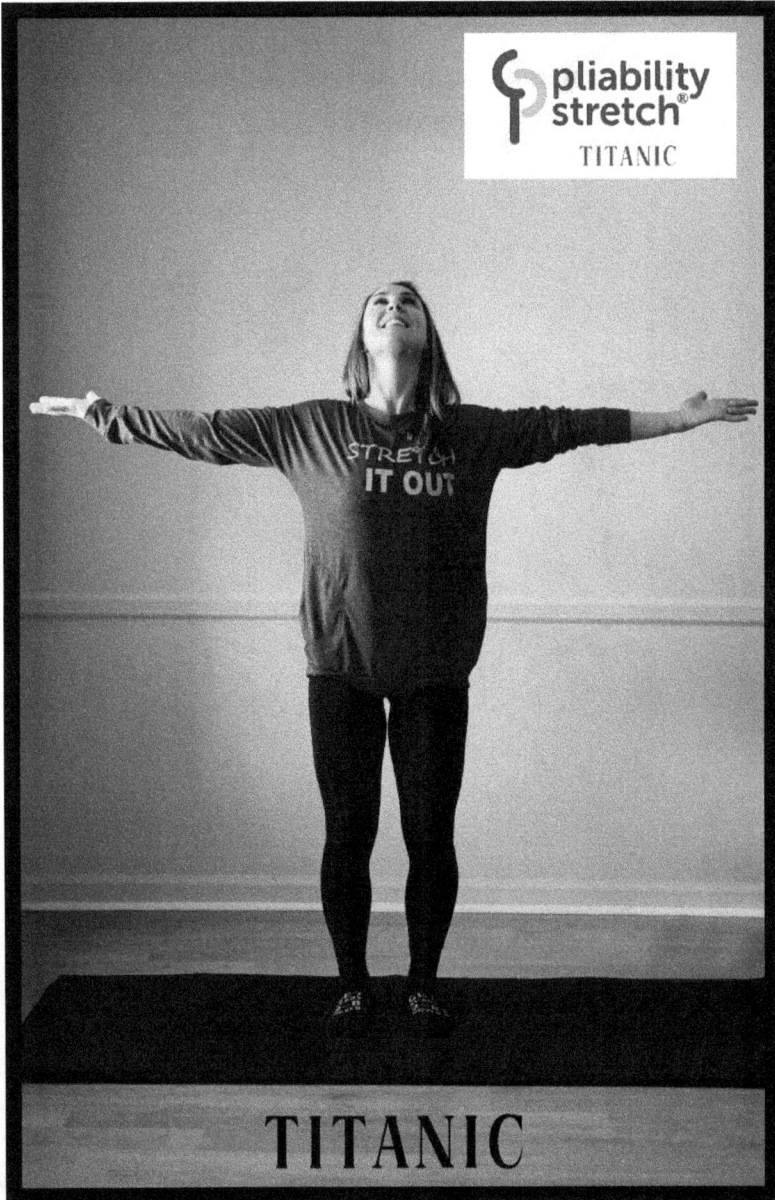

Assisted Stretch Technique

- Place your hands around the side of the client's cervical neck like a hammock. Cue client to take a breath in
- Cue the client to inhale and on the exhale to lift the chin and chest to the ceiling.
- Gently increase the cervical extension stretch

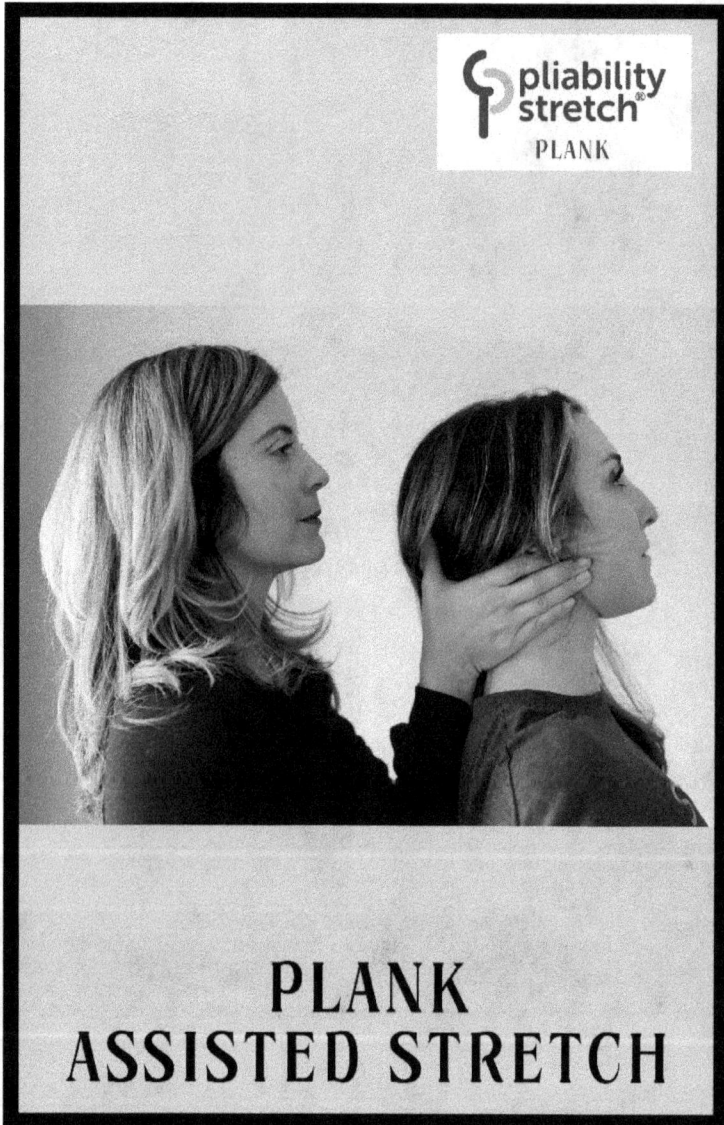

PLANK
ASSISTED STRETCH

ZIPPER DOWN INTO FORWARD FOLD
Stretch Technique

- Cue client to drop the chin to the chest and continue to roll-down until they touch the floor. (Executed while sitting on a chair for clients with mobility limitations.)
- Cue client to bend knees and drop the buttocks in order to reach the floor.
- Ask client to hold in forward fold position.
- Add manual stretch of torso to legs.

*If client is unable to zipper to the floor then exclude remaining warm up.

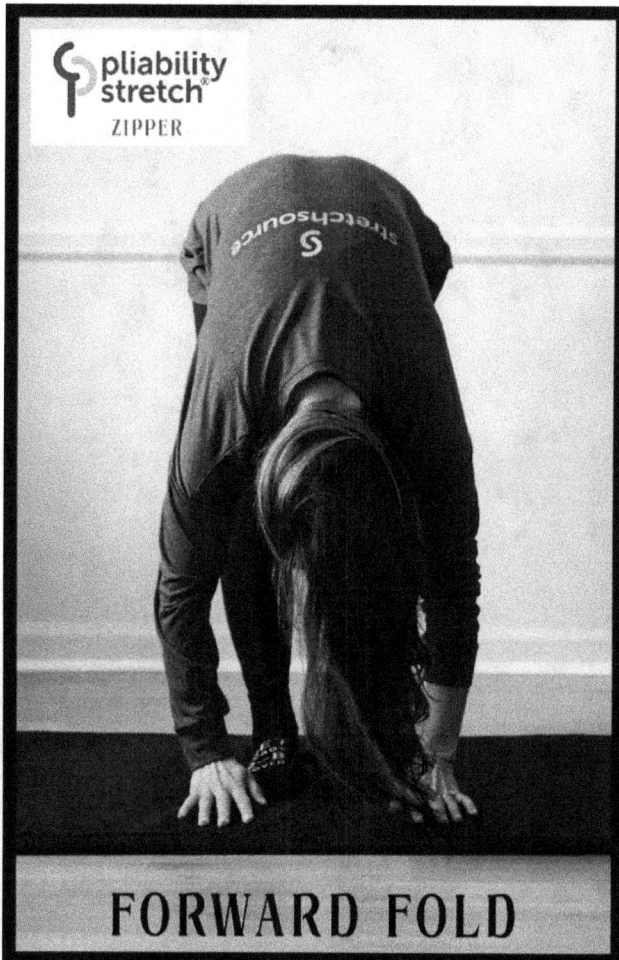

FORWARD FOLD

Assisted Stretch Technique
- While the client is forward folded, place your arms at the bra line and above the knees.
- As the client exhales, gently press your arms together to increase the stretch.

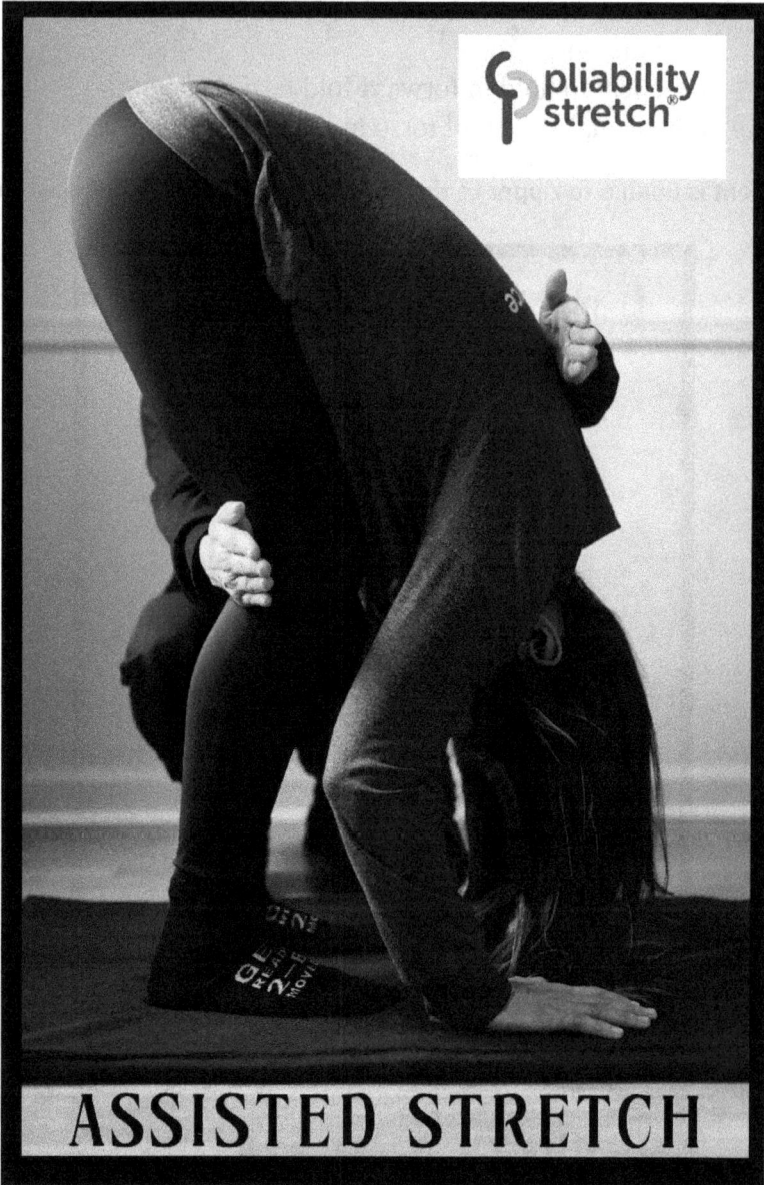

ASSISTED STRETCH

PLANK
Stretch Technique
- Cue client during exhale to walk out to a plank position with proper form.
- Add manual stretch of calves and ankles.

*If wrist pain is present with plank, then modify to forearms and exclude downward dog.

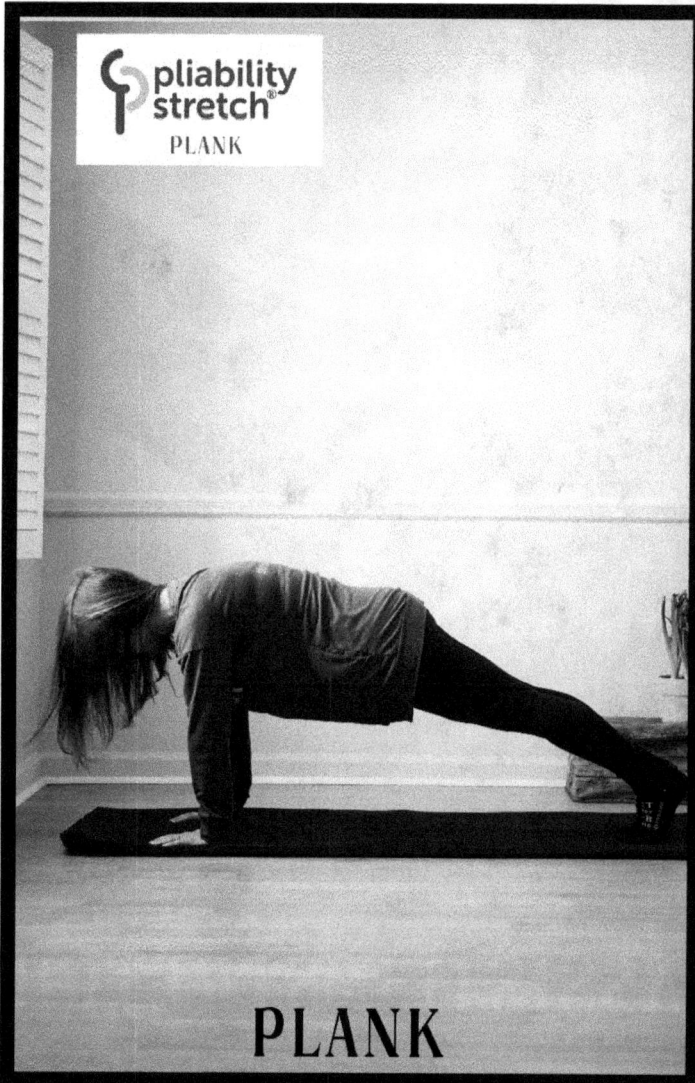

Assisted Stretch Technique
- Place your hands on the back of the client's ankles
- Gentle increase the stretch to the achilles

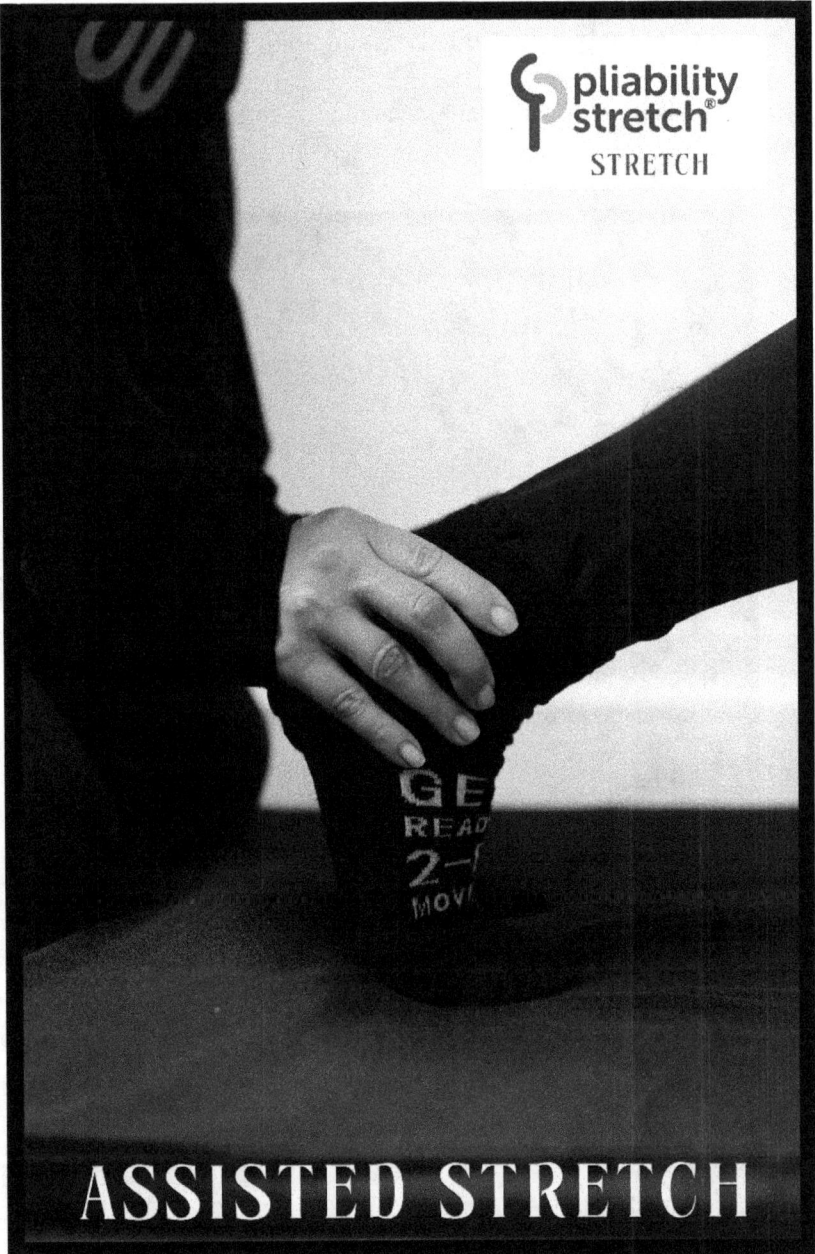

ASSISTED STRETCH

DOWNWARD DOG
Stretch Technique

- Cue your client during exhale to keep hands where they are and to push back into downward dog. (Use wall for a client with mobility limitations).
- Add 3 different manual stretches. (external, medial, achilles)

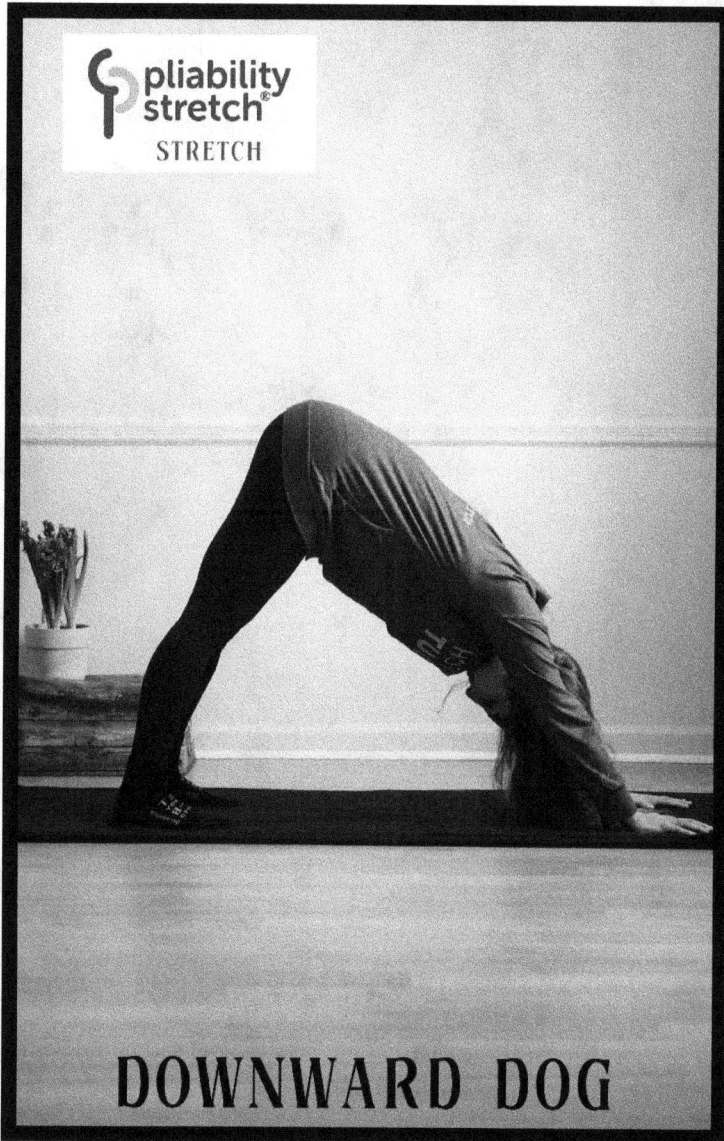

DOWNWARD DOG

Assisted Stretch Technique
- Place your hands on the outside of the legs and above the knees.
- Gently sit your weight back to increase the stretch

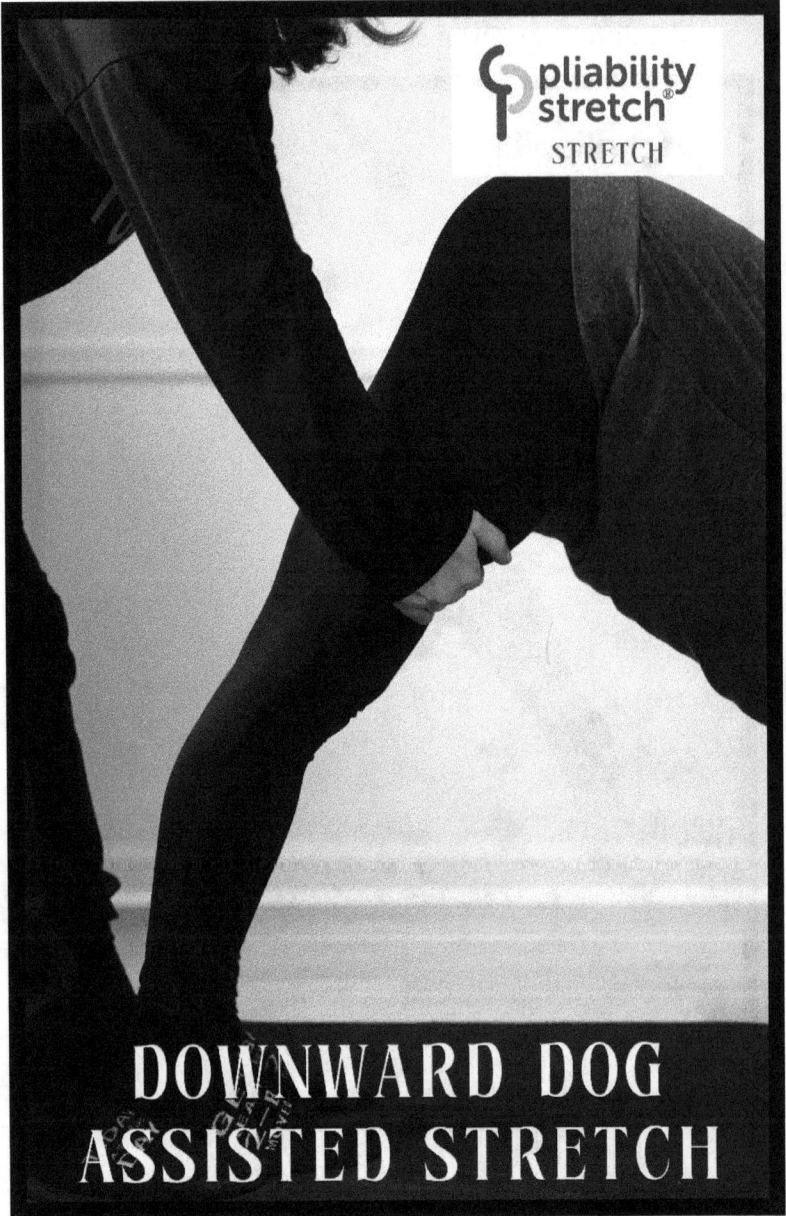

DOWNWARD DOG ASSISTED STRETCH

CHILD POSE

Stretch Technique

- Cue your client to sit back onto feet while keeping hands stationary. (Placing arms by the side or under the head can be considered for clients with mobility limitations as well as a rolled up towel under their buttocks).

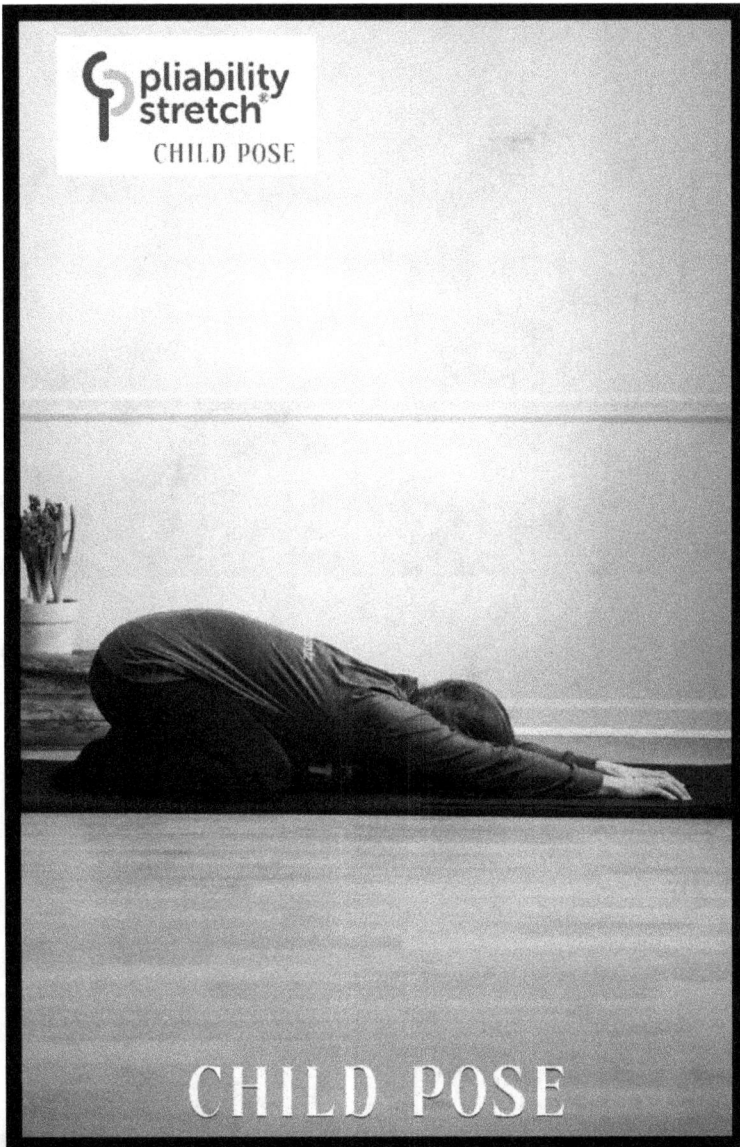

Assisted Stretch Technique

- Gently press on the lower back for relief

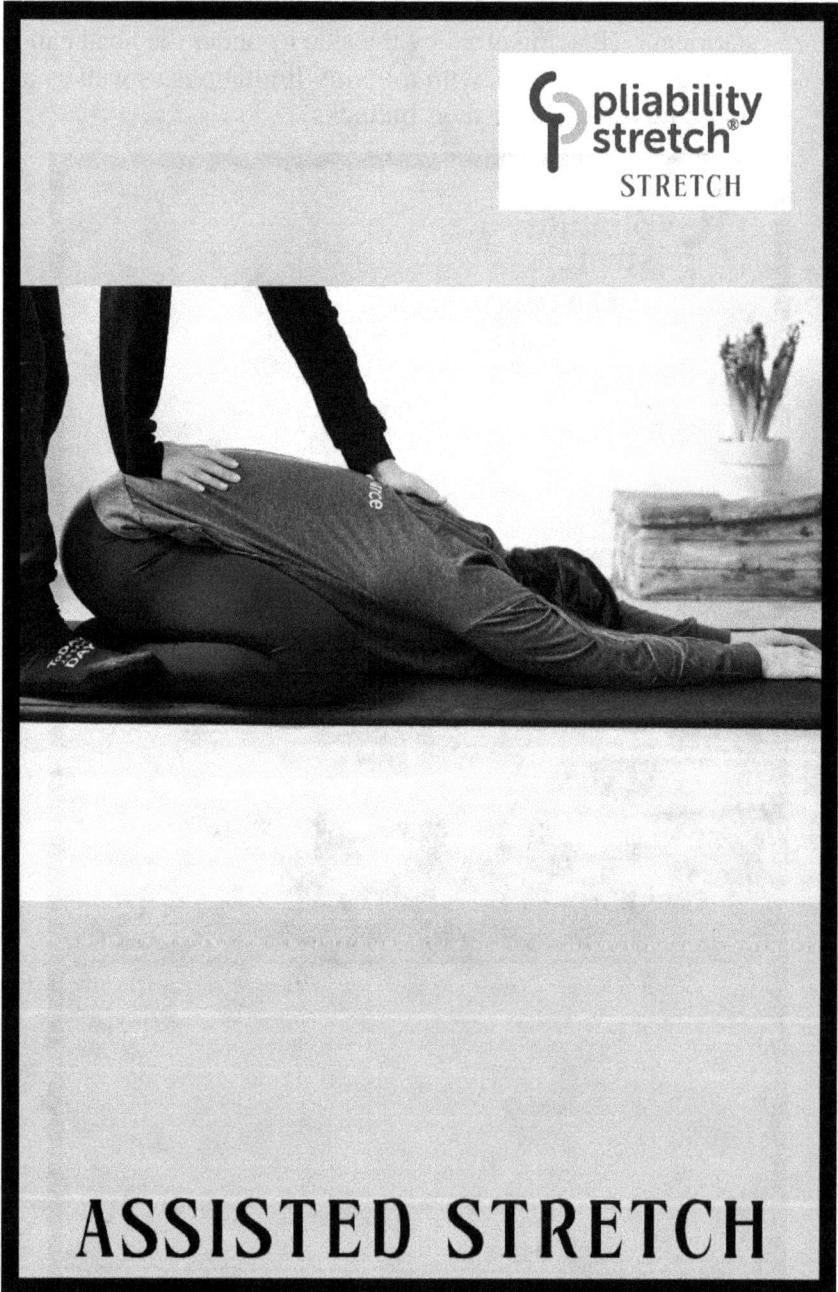

ASSISTED STRETCH

ALL FOURS TO FORWARD FOLD
Stretch Technique

- Cue your client to return to all fours, tuck toes under, walk hands back to knees and then lift knees up and continue walking back into forward fold.

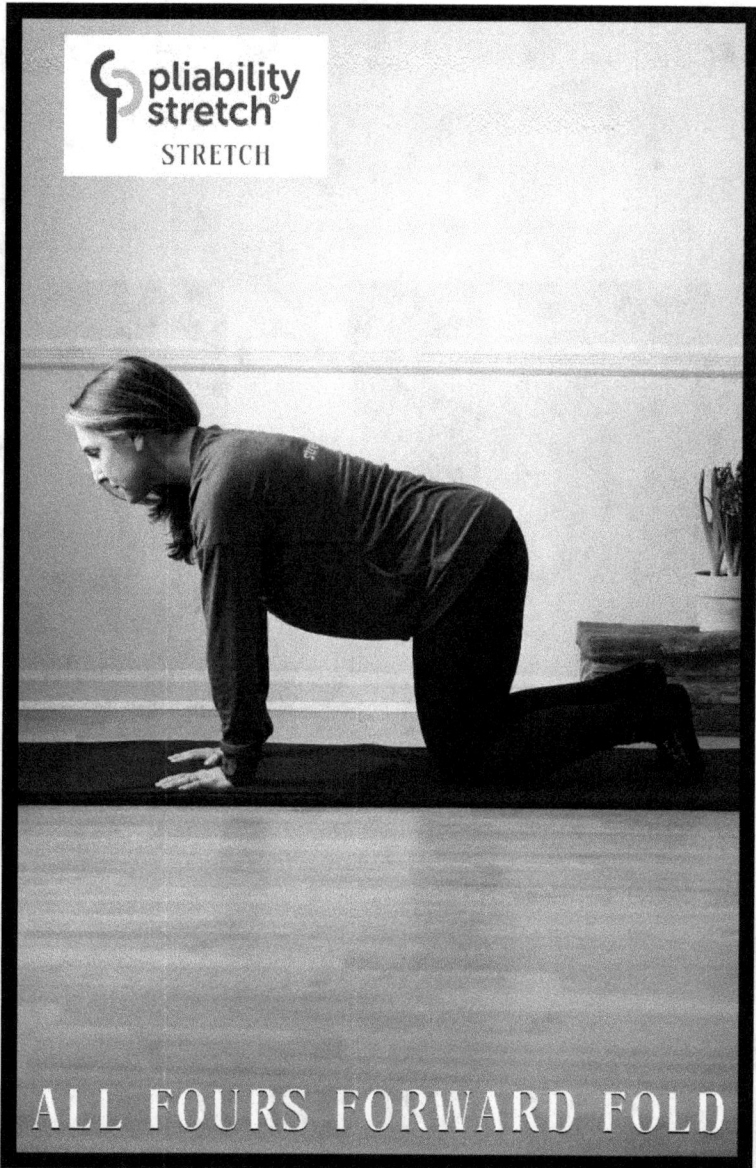

ALL FOURS FORWARD FOLD

Zipper Up
Stretch Technique

- Once forward fold is established then cue the client to roll back up with head arriving last.

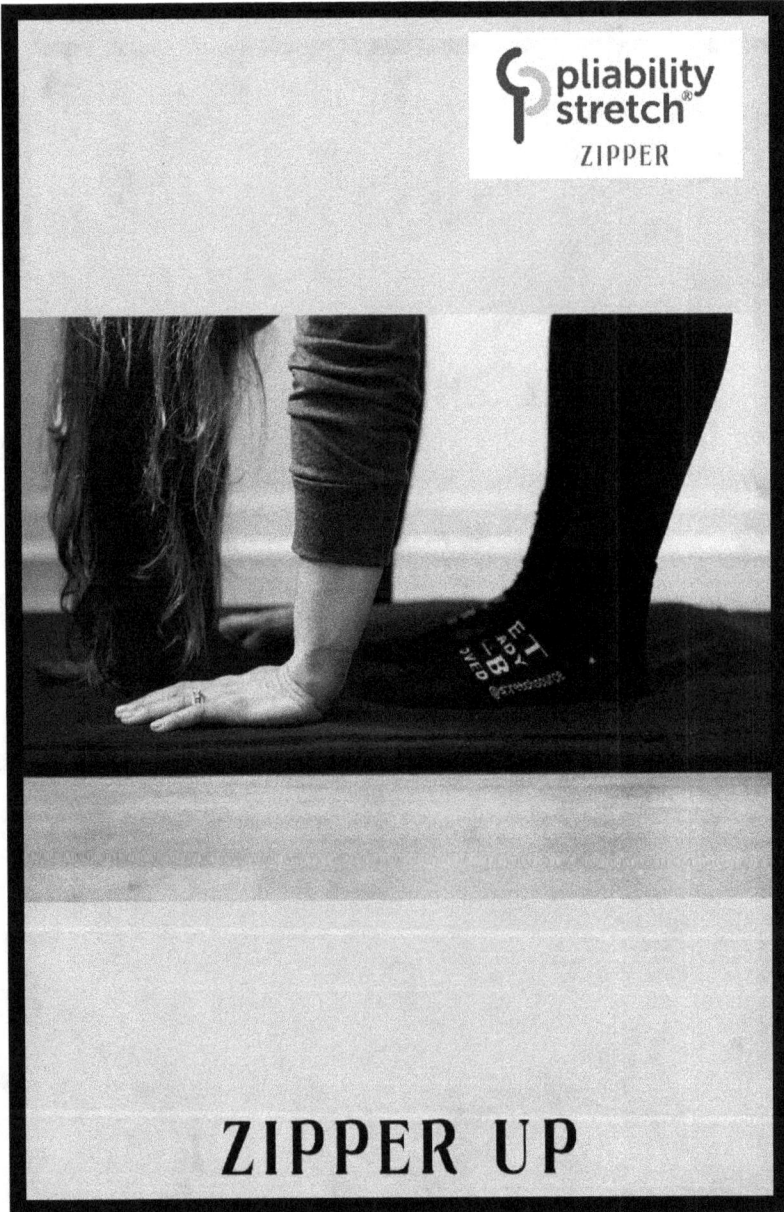

Section 2

Chapter 3
The Stretch Series

1. Series I

2. Series II

3. Series III

4. Series IV

SERIES I

A client remains lying supine throughout this series. Constantly remind the client of the need for open communication and continue breathing. If a client is feeling any stretch in an area other than where they should, then the following should be considered:

- Is the client completely relaxed and the complete weight of the stretch in the trainer's control?
- Is the joint being stretched and stabilized appropriately or moving to cause the client unnecessary discomfort and strain?
- Is the client engaging muscles during the stretch?
- Can the trainer stabilize the joint more effectively?

* Client may need head support.

Series 1

Hamstring
Cross-Over
Adductor

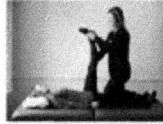

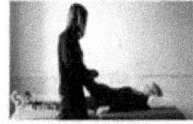

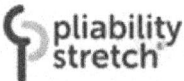

pliability
stretch

Single Lumbar Press
Hip Circle - Rotator
Hip Circle – Single Twist

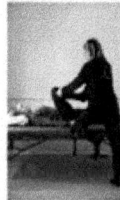

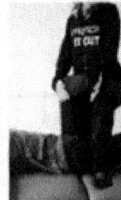

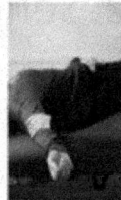

HAMSTRING
Stretch Technique
- The client's legs are straight and aligned with hips.
- Begin with one straight leg. Slowly raise the leg to the ceiling. Check the standing leg for positioning and place your knee on the thigh for stabilization.
- Ask the client to communicate when a stretch is felt.
- Continue pressing deeper into the stretch until the client communicates a feeling of a nice amount of stretching.
- Hold the position for 15-30 seconds.
- Add a flex of the foot for calf stretch.
- Repeat on the other leg.

Muscles being stretched
Primary muscles: semimembranosus, semitendinosus, biceps femoris
Secondary muscle: gastrocnemius

Injuries where stretch may be useful:
lower back muscle strain, lower back ligament sprain, hamstring strain, calf strain

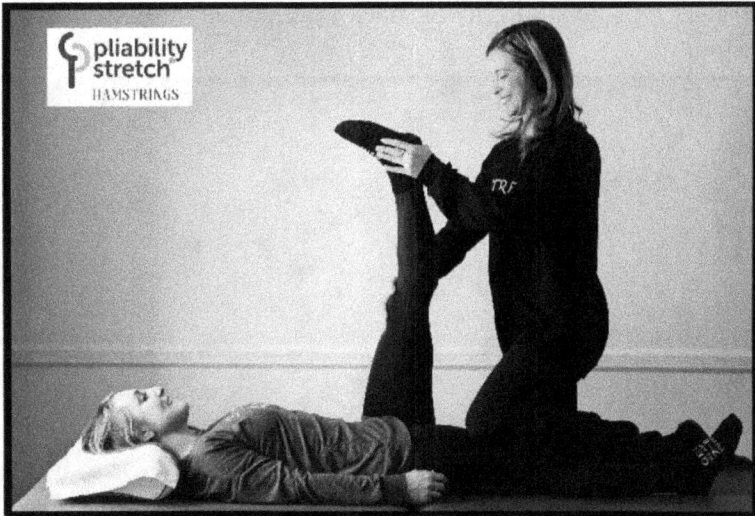

CROSS-OVER (IT band- iliotibial band)
Stretch Technique
- The client's legs are straight and aligned with hips.
- Begin with one straight leg. Slowly cross the leg over the other leg and continue to side raise the leg across the client's body.
- Ask the client to communicate when a stretch is felt.
- Continue pressing deeper into the stretch until the client communicates a feeling of a nice amount of stretching.
- Hold the position for 15-30 seconds.
- Add a soleus stretch by rotating the foot in and out.
- Repeat on the other leg.

Muscles being stretched
Primary muscles: semispinalis thoracic, spinalis thoracis, longissimus thoracis, iliocostalis thoracis, iliocostalis lumborum, multifidus, rotators, intertransversarii, interspines
Secondary muscles: gluteus maximus, medius and minimus, tensor fasciae latae

Injuries where stretch may be useful:
lower back muscle strain, lower back ligament sprain, iliotibial band syndrome

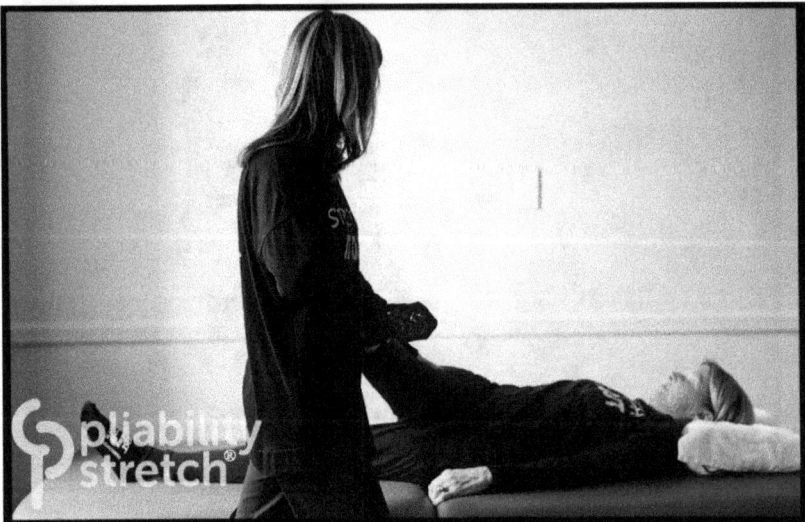

ADDUCTOR

Stretch Technique

- The client's legs straight and aligned with hips.
- Begin with one straight leg. Slowly raise the leg to the side of the body. Check the pelvis to make sure both hips are remaining in position on the table. Adjust leg height as needed. Stabilize standing leg with your thigh and working leg with your opposite knee. Your position is similar to a lunge.
- Ask the client to communicate when he/she feels a stretch.
- Continue pressing deeper into the stretch until the client communicates a feeling of a nice amount of stretching.
- Hold the position for 15-30 seconds.
- Repeat on the other leg.

Muscles being stretched

Primary muscles: adductor longus, brevis, and magnus.
Secondary muscles: gracilis. pectineus, Semimembronasus, semitendinosus

Injuries where stretch may be useful:

groin strain, osteitis pubis, piriformis syndrome, tendonitis of the adductor muscles, trochanteric bursitis. hamstring strain

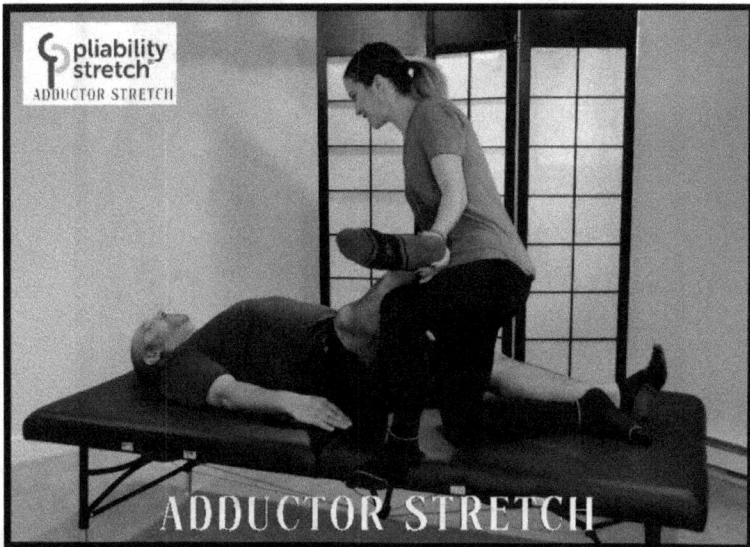

SINGLE LUMBAR PRESS

Stretch Technique
- Bend the client's legs. Grab both knees and bring the client's knees towards the chest.
- Ask the client to communicate when he/she feels a stretch.
- Continue pressing deeper into the stretch until the client communicates a feeling of a nice amount of stretching.
- Hold the position for 15-30 seconds.
- Repeat on the other leg.

Muscles being stretched
Primary muscles: gluteus maximus
Secondary muscles: iliocostalis lumborum, spinalis thoracis, longissimus thoracis

Injuries where stretch may be useful:
lower back muscle strain, lower back ligament sprain, hamstring strain

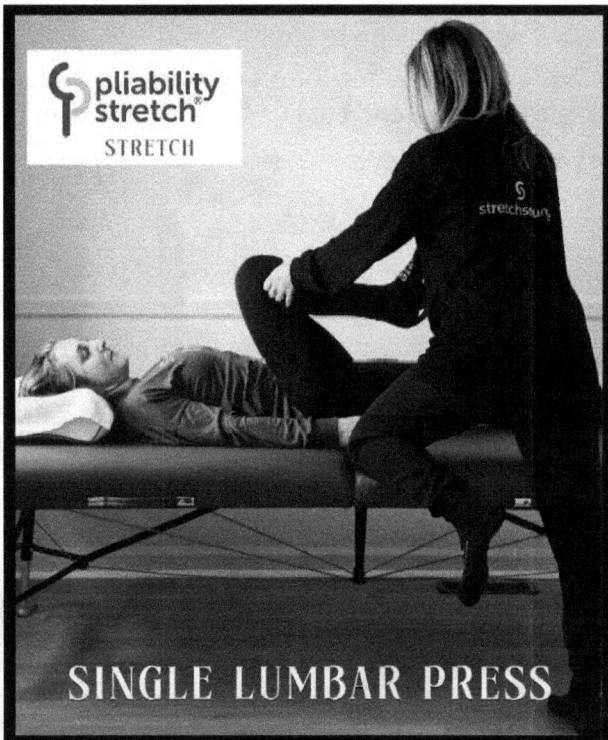

SINGLE LUMBAR PRESS

HIP ROTATOR
Stretch Technique
- Client is positioned with legs straight.
- Bend one knee and raise it to hip height. Slowly rotate the bent knee to external hip rotation.
- Ask the client to communicate when he/she feels a stretch.
- Continue pressing deeper until the client communicates a feeling of a nice amount of stretching or the knee ankle alignment becomes 90 degrees.
- Continue deeper into stretch if the client desires by pressing the bent position into the client's chest.
- Ask the client to communicate when he/she feels a stretch.
- Continue pressing deeper into the stretch until the client communicates a feeling of a nice amount of stretching.
- Hold the position for 15-30 seconds.
- Repeat on the other leg.

Muscles being stretched
Primary muscles: piriformis, gemellus superior and inferior, obsturator internus and externus, quadratus femoris
Secondary muscles: gluteus maximus

Injuries where stretch may be useful:
piriformis syndrome, snapping hip syndrome, trochanteric bursitis

HIP CIRCLES ROTATOR

SINGLE TWIST
Stretch Technique
- Client is positioned with legs straight.
- Bend one knee and raise to hip height.
- Circle knee without compressing on the hip joint.
- Take knee over opposite side.
- Add arm extension for additional chest, shoulder stretch.

Muscles being stretched
Primary muscles: lower back
Secondary muscles: shoulders

Injuries where stretch may be useful:
sciatica. menstrual discomfort, digestive issues, upper back pain and neck pain

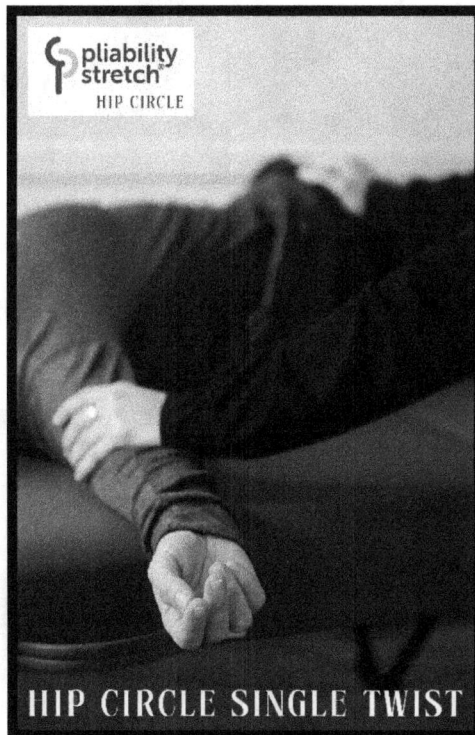

SERIES II

A client is instructed to roll onto his/her side into a chair position. He/she may place the under arm into a comfortable position. A towel can be used to increase the comfort of the head in this position. Check that the client is lying with good alignment and a relaxed/comfortable position.

pliability stretch® Series 2

| Shoulder Activation | Reach | Book Opener | Forward Hamstring | Reverse Quad |

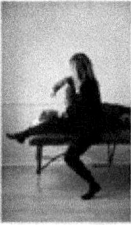 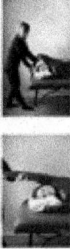 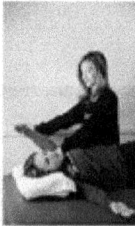 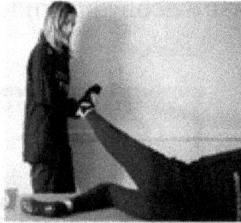 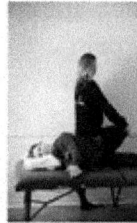

SHOUDER ACTIVATION AND LATERAL REACH
Stretch Technique

- Taking just the top arm, hook the client's elbow into trainer's elbow.
- Position the shoulder joint into appropriate alignment and stabilize with trainer's free other hand.
- Gently circle the elbow. Increase the diameter of the circle each time until the client communicates a nice stretch.
- Reverse the circle.
- Stretch arm long over-head while stabilizing shoulder.

Muscles being stretched
Primary muscles: trapezius
Secondary muscles: deltoid, pectoralis, serratus, scapulae, rhomboids

Injuries where stretch may be useful:
frozen shoulder, neck pain, shoulder pain, shoulder bursitis

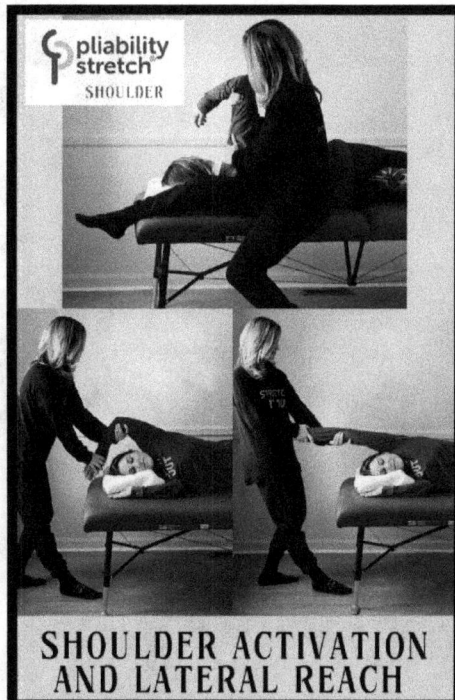

SHOULDER ACTIVATION AND LATERAL REACH

BOOK OPENER

Stretch Technique

- Place client's arms straight out on table
- With an exhale lift top arm to ceiling and over to opposing side of the body
- Ask the client to communicate when he/she feel a stretch
- Repeat 2x

Muscles being stretched

Primary muscles: lower back
Secondary muscles: Shoulders

Injuries where stretch may be useful:

Sciatica, menstrual discomfort, digestive issues, upper back pain and neck pain

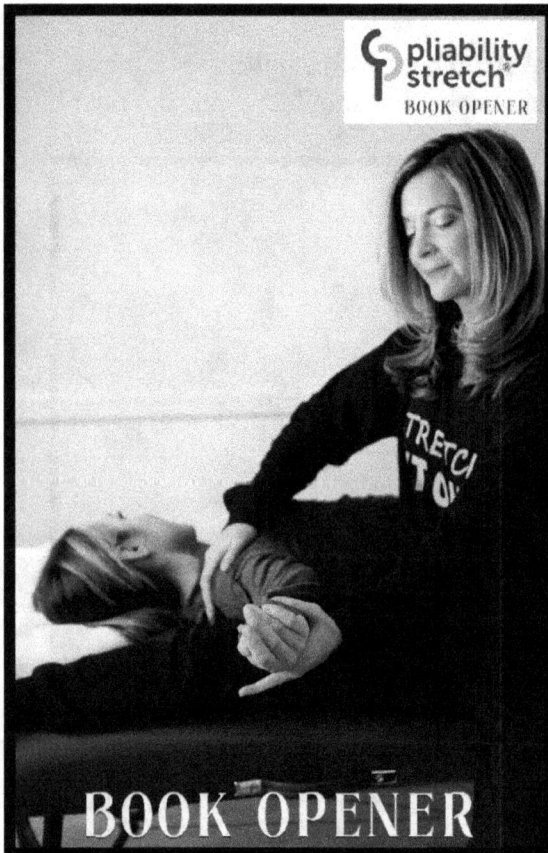

FORWARD HAMSTRING
Stretch Technique
- Straighten just the top leg to the end of the table.
- Raise the leg in line with the hip.
- Slowly bring the leg forward while stabilizing the standing leg with your thigh or hand.
- Ask the client to communicate to you when he/she feels a stretch.
- Continue pressing deeper into the stretch until the client communicates a feeling of a nice amount of stretching.
- Hold the position for 15-30 seconds.

Muscles being stretched
Primary muscle: gluteus maximus
Secondary muscle: semimembranosus, semitendinosus, biceps femoris

Injuries where stretch may be useful:
lower back muscle strain, lower back ligament sprain, hamstring sprain, iliotibial band syndrome

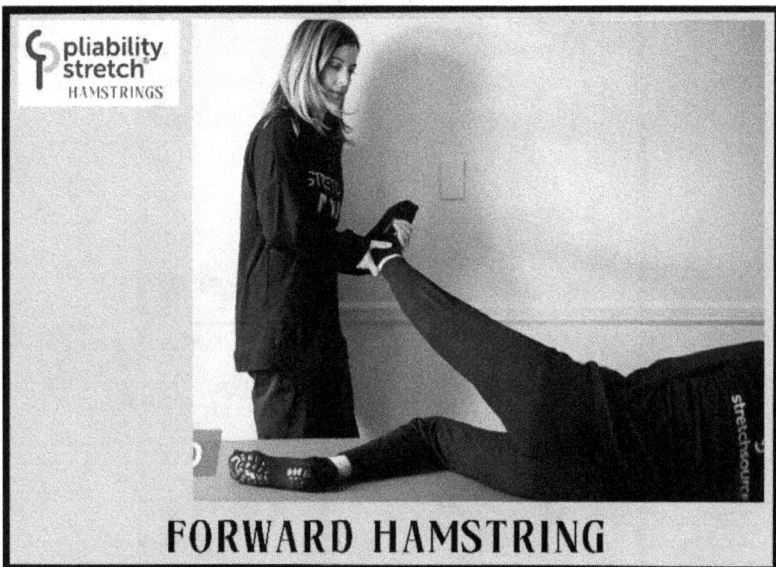

FORWARD HAMSTRING

REVERSE QUAD
Stretch Technique
- Take the top leg and bend it back into a 90-degree angle.
- Continue to pull the leg behind the client for a quad stretch. Ask the client to communicate to you when they feel a stretch.
- Continue pressing deeper into the stretch until the client communicates a feeling of a nice amount of stretching.
- Hold the position for 15-30 seconds.

Muscles being stretched
Primary muscle: rectus femoris, vastus medialis, lateralis and intermedius
Secondary muscle: iliacus. psoas major

Injuries where stretch may be useful:
hip flexor strain, ostetis pubis, iliopsoas tendonitis, trochanteric bursitis, quadriceps strain, quadriceps tendonitis, patellofemoral pain syndrome, patellar tendonitis, subluxing kneecap

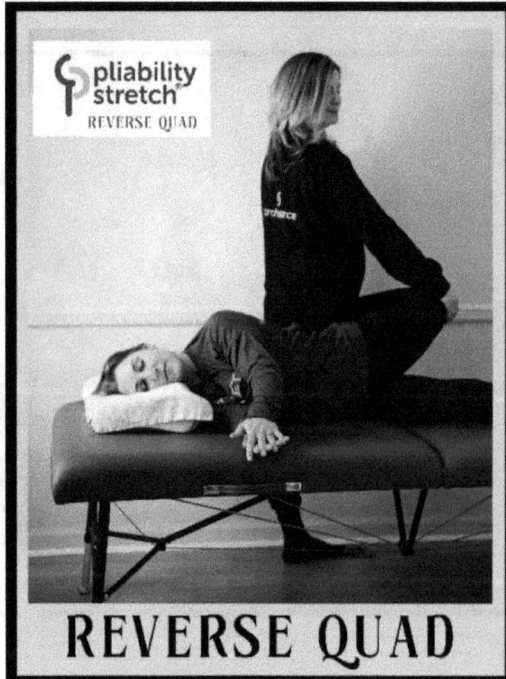

REVERSE QUAD

Series III

Ask the to come to a sitting position on the edge of the table with feet placed aligned to hips. General rule of thumb is to find the degree of stretch that is comfortable for the client and hold for 15-30 seconds. client

Series 3

T-twist
Scapular Protraction
Chest Expansion
Triceps
Cross Body Shoulder
Forward Fold
Neck Series
Chest Opener – Forward Fold
Psoas

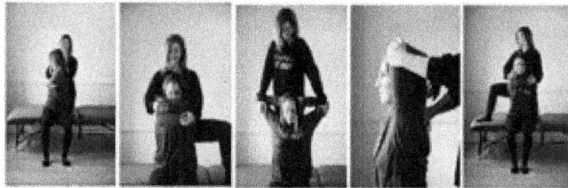

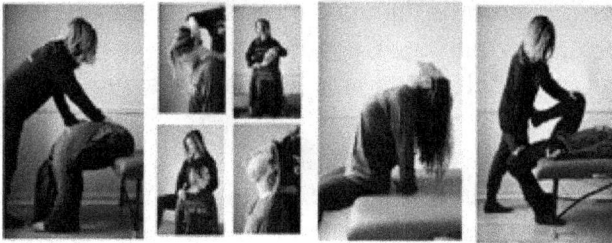

pliability
stretch

T-TWIST
Stretch Technique
- Client sits upright at the edge of the table with feet on the floor and arms extended into t-shape.
- Instruct the client to twist in one direction with exhaling breath.
- Guide the stretch further by pushing against the upper back and pulling on cross body shoulder.
- Instruct the client to return to neutral with an inhale breath and twist other direction with exhale.
- Repeat as needed.

Muscles being stretched
Primary muscle: semispinalis thoracis, spinalis thoracis, longissimus thoracis, iliocostalis thoracis, iliocostalis lumborum, multifidus, rotatores, intertranversarii, interspinales
Secondary muscle: quadratus lumborum, external and internal obliques.

Injuries where stretch may be useful:
back muscle strain, back ligament sprain, abdominal muscle strain(obliques).

pliability
stretch®
STRETCH

T-TWIST
ASSISTED STRETCH

Scapular Protraction
Stretch Technique
- Client sits upright and hugs arms across body with shoulder in proper position (no alleviated shoulders).
- On exhale pull client's elbows into scapular protraction.
- Hold stretch for 30 seconds.

Muscles being stretched
Primary muscle: rhomboids, scapular
Secondary muscle: triceps

Injuries where stretch may be useful:
Neck and shoulder pain

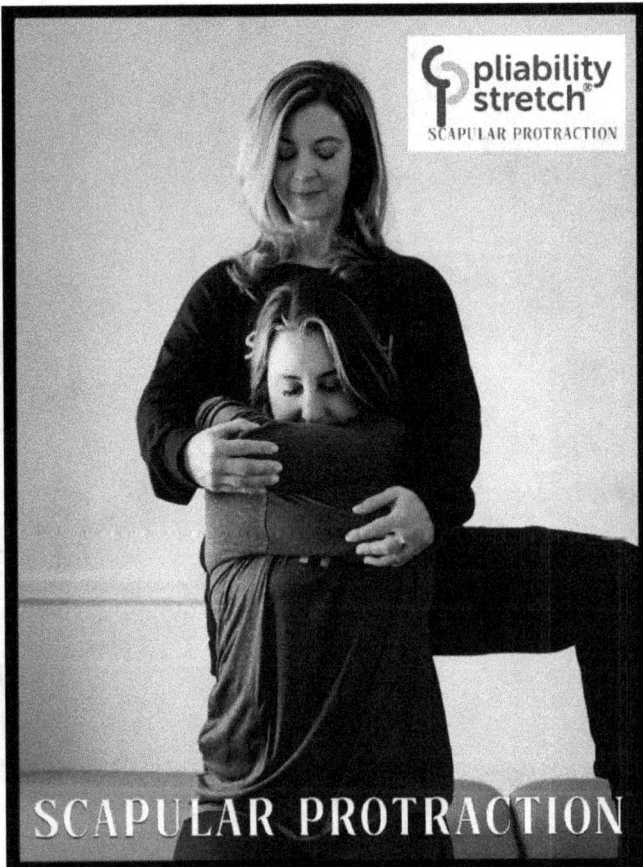

CHEST EXPANSION

Stretch Technique

- Ask client to clasp fingers and place behind head with elbows close together. Check for shoulder alignment and adjust position as needed.
- Place yourself up against the client's back for stabilization.
- Take an elbow into each hand and slowly pull the elbows apart.
- Ask the client to communicate to you when a stretch is felt.

Muscles being stretched

Primary muscle: pectoral major and minor
Secondary muscle: shoulders

Injuries where stretch may be useful:
neck and shoulder

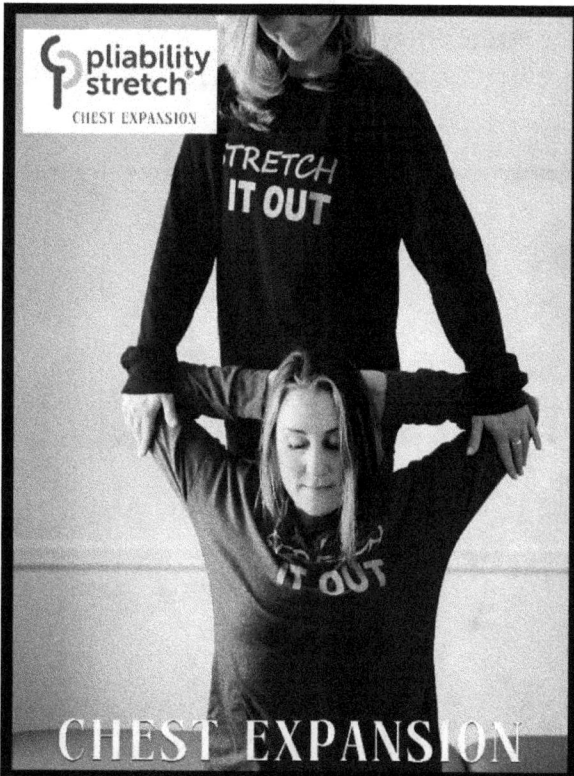

Triceps
Stretch Technique

- Keep one hand behind the head and drop another arm to the table.
- Pin the hand to the shoulder with a dropped elbow.
- Hold the pinned hand and use other hand to gently raise the elbow.
- Ask the client to communicate to you when they feel a stretch.
- Continue pressing deeper into the stretch until the client communicates a feeling of a nice amount of stretching.
- Hold the position for 15-30 seconds.

Muscles being stretched

Primary muscle: triceps brachii
Secondary muscle: latissimus dorsi, teres major and minor.

Injuries where stretch may be useful:

elbow sprain, elbow dislocation elbow bursitis. triceps tendon rupture.

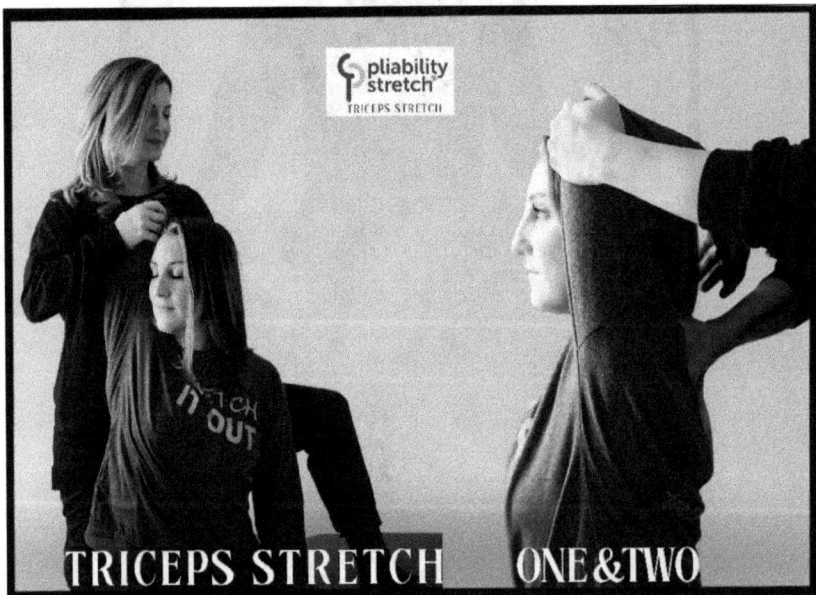

CROSS BODY SHOULDER
Stretch Technique

- Take one arm out to the side and then across the client's body until the hand reaches the opposite shoulder.
- Check for shoulder alignment.
- Hold the hand-free shoulder down as you pull the elbow away.
- Ask the client to communicate to you when a stretch is felt.
- Continue pressing deeper into the stretch until the client communicates a feeling of a nice amount of stretching.
- Hold the position for 15-30 seconds.

Muscles being stretched
Primary muscle: trapezius, rhomboids, latissimus dorsi, posterior deltoid

Secondary muscle: infraspinatus, teres minor.

Injuries where stretch may be useful:
Dislocation, impingement syndrome, rotator cuff tendonitis, shoulder bursitis, frozen shoulder

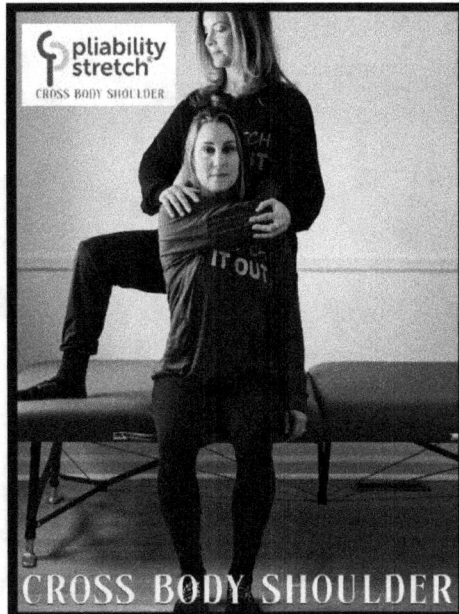

FORWARD FOLD

Stretch Technique

- Have client clasp hands behind their back, open chest and look up to the ceiling.
- Have client drop the chin and fold over legs with head to the ground and hands reach to the ceiling for a desired stretch.
- Let them hold the position briefly and then ask them to unclasp hands as you take one hand and then the other and the hands to the floor.
- Allow the client to remain in forward fold.
- Apply pressure to the back for extra stretch.
- Ask client to roll-up with the head stacking up last.

Muscles being stretched

Primary muscle: anterior deltoid
Secondary muscle: biceps brachii, brachialis., coracobrachialis

Injuries where stretch may be useful:

impingement syndrome, rotator cuff tendonitis, shoulder bursitis, frozen shoulder, chest strain., pectoral muscle insertion inflammation

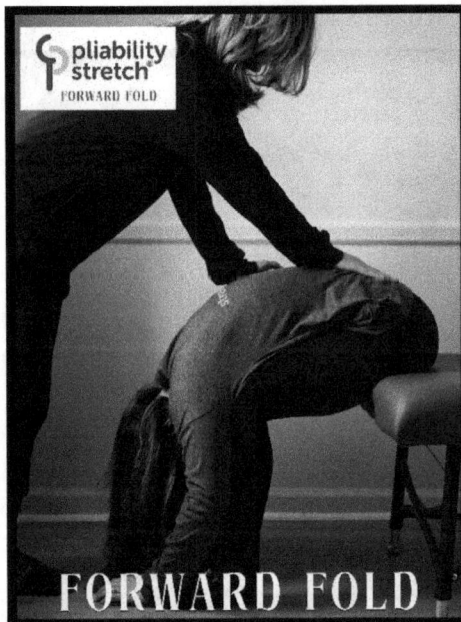

NECK

Stretch Technique

- Stretching the neck from ear to shoulder right and left while stabilizing the shoulder.
- Stretching the neck down chin to chest and up chin to ceiling while holding the weight of the head throughout.
- Stretching the neck by rotating the nose right and left while stabilizing the shoulder.
- Always ask the client for feedback.

Muscles being stretched

Lateral Bend primary muscle: levator scapula, trapezius

Rotating primary muscle: sternocleidomastoideus, Forward flexion primary muscle: semispinalis capitis and cervices, spinalis capitis and cervices, longissimus capitis and cervicis, splenius capitis and cervicis

Neck extension primary muscle: platysma and sternocleidomastoid

Injuries where stretch may be useful:
Neck muscle strain, whiplash, cervical nerve stretch syndrome, wryneck

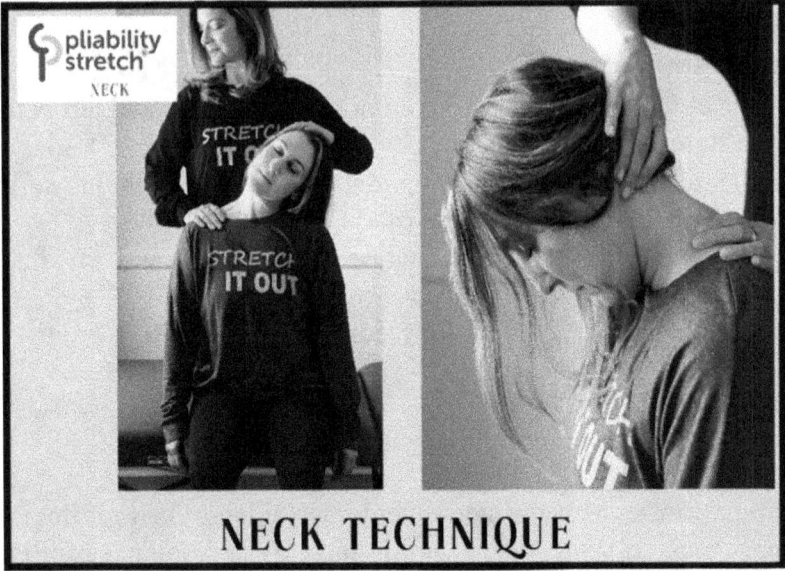

NECK TECHNIQUE

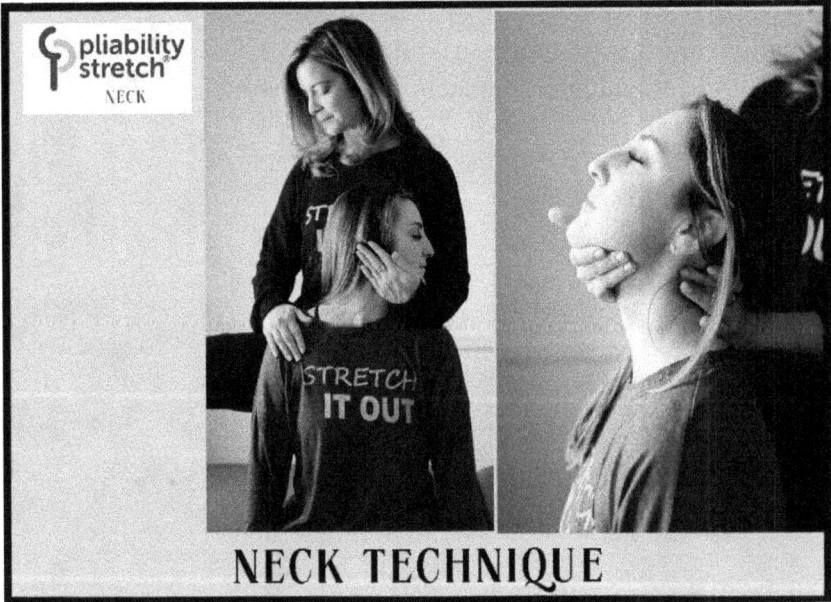

NECK TECHNIQUE

CHEST OPENER AND FORWARD FOLD
Stretch Technique
- Client clasps hands behind back and opens chest to ceiling.
- Instruct client to take position into forward fold and then release hands.
- Instruct client to release and relax in forward fold and then zipper back up to sitting position.
- Continue pressing deeper into the stretch until the client communicates a feeling of a nice amount of stretching.
- Hold the position for 15-30 seconds.

Muscles being stretched
Primary muscle: pectoralis major and minor, anterior deltoid
Secondary muscle: serratus anterior

Injuries where stretch may be useful:
impingement syndrome, rotator cuff tendonitis, shoulder bursitis, frozen shoulder, chest strain, pectoral muscle insertion inflammation.

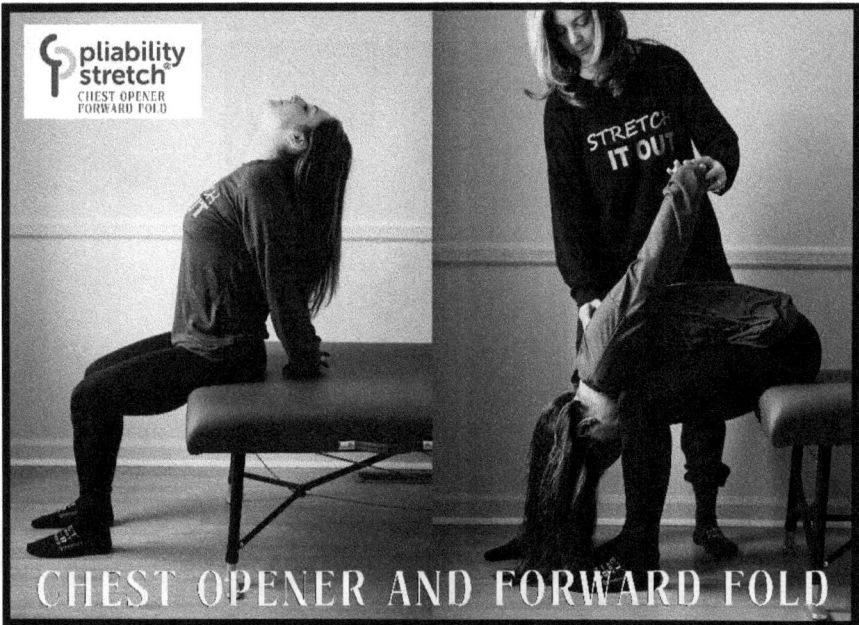

CHEST OPENER AND FORWARD FOLD

PSOAS

Stretch Technique

- Have client sit on the very edge of the table.
- Ask client to hold one knee to his/her chest and guide client to lie back onto the table.
- Align the client on the table and all the joints.
- Increase stretch as needed by moving the foot back and then up.
- If there is any discomfort in areas other than the psoas and quad then assess and stabilize joint.

Muscles being stretched

Primary muscles: rectus femoris, vastus medialis, lateralis, and intermedius
Secondary muscles: iliacus, psoas major

Injuries where stretch may be useful:

hip flexor straining, osteitis pubis, iliopsoas tendonitis, trochanteric bursitis, quadriceps tendonitis, patellofemoral pain syndrome, patellar tendonitis, subluxing kneecap

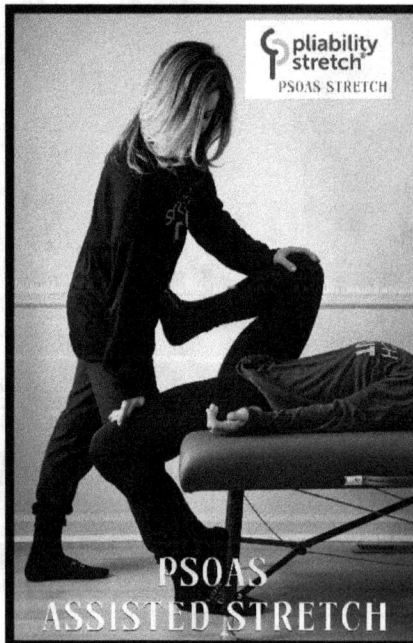

SERIES IV

Series IV is about bringing the body to rest after all the intense stretching. At this point in the session the client should feel like a whole new person and walk away feeling like a million bucks.

Series 4

pliability stretch

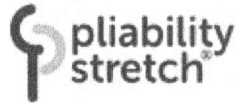

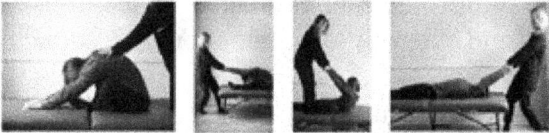

Butterfly
Assisted Roll-Down
Release and Relax
Wrist and Fingers
Ankle Stretch

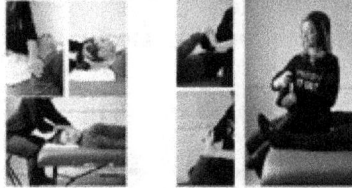

BUTTERFLY
Stretch Technique
- Ask client to sit in the middle of the table with legs in butterfly position.
- Have the client stretch forward over legs.
- Press gently on the thighs to desired stretch.
- Press gently on the back for desired stretch.
- Ask the client to roll-up with the head arriving last.

Muscles being stretched
Primary muscles: piriformis, gemellus superior and inferior, obturator internus and externus, quadratus femoris, adductor longus, brevis and magnus
Secondary muscles: gluteus maximus, gracilis, pectineus

Injuries where stretch may be useful:
Piriformis syndrome. Groin strain. Tendonitis of the adductor muscles. Snapping hip syndrome. Trochanteric bursitis.

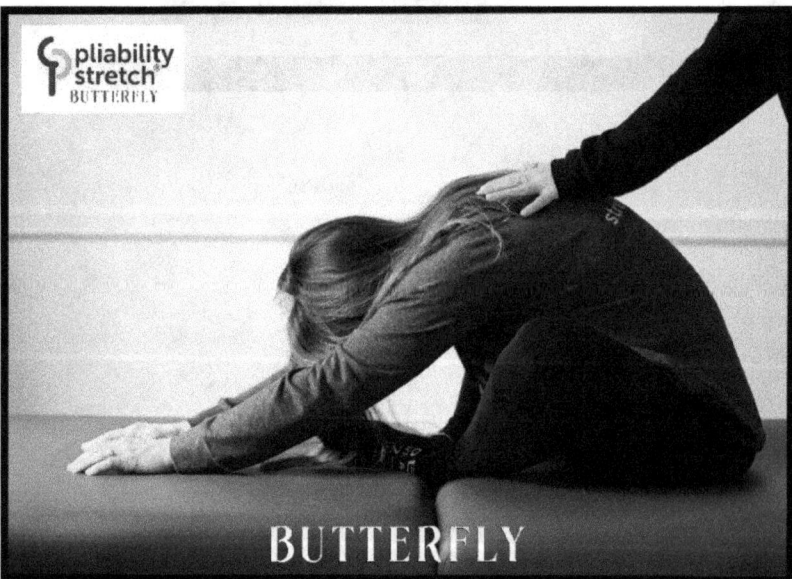
BUTTERFLY

ASSISTED ROLL-DOWN
Stretch Technique

- Client is lying supine with legs straight.
- Take hold of the client's wrist.
- Ask client to tuck chin, lean back to the table and allow the trainer to slowly lower them down.
- Ask client to keep arms reaching to ceiling.
- On exhale pull arms over head for full body stretch and torso elongation.
- Retrograde back to sitting up and repeat as needed.

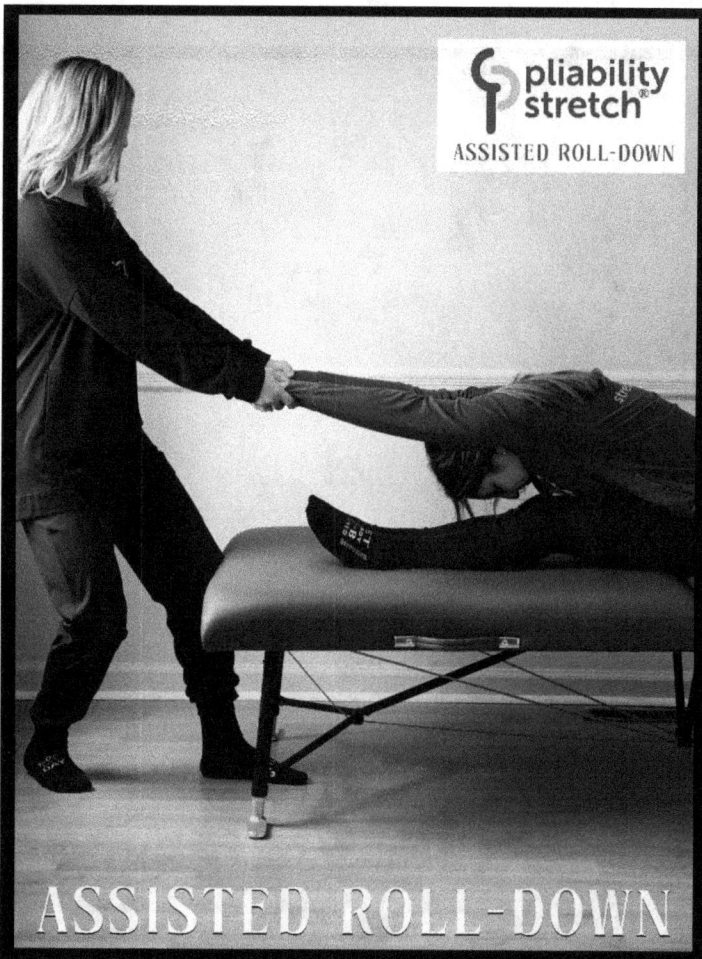

RELEASE AND RELAX
Stretch Technique
- Client is lying supine with arms by side and legs straight. (provide pillow under knees if needed)
- Manipulate neck until you reach the base where the spine meets the skull.
- Gentle traction of the neck.
- Gentle lift of head off the table and into extension.
- Side neck stretch (L/R)
- Twist neck stretch (L/R)
- Chest press

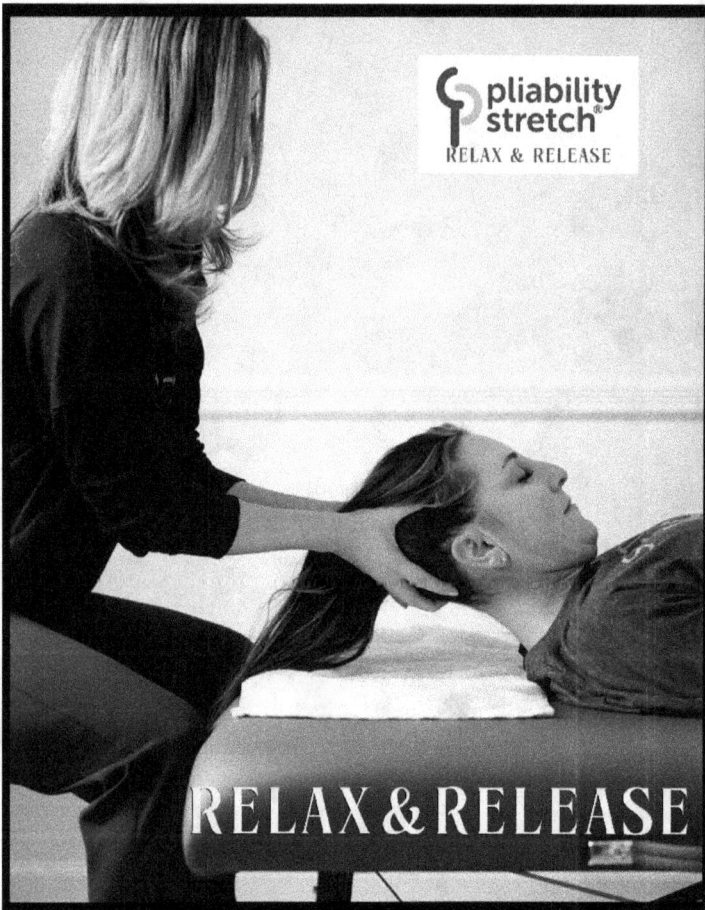

pliability
stretch®
RELAX

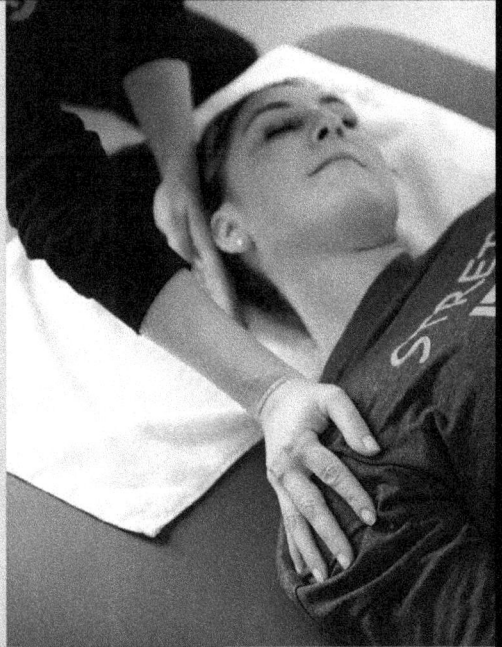

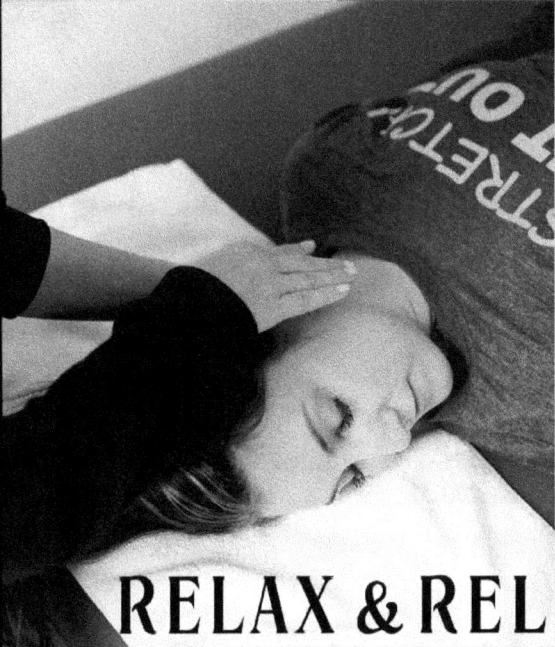

RELAX & RELEASE

WRIST AND FINGERS

Technique

- Interlace trainer and client fingers with client's arm straight.
- Bend the wrist up for desired stretch.
- Bend the wrist down for desired stretch.
- Always ask the client for feedback.

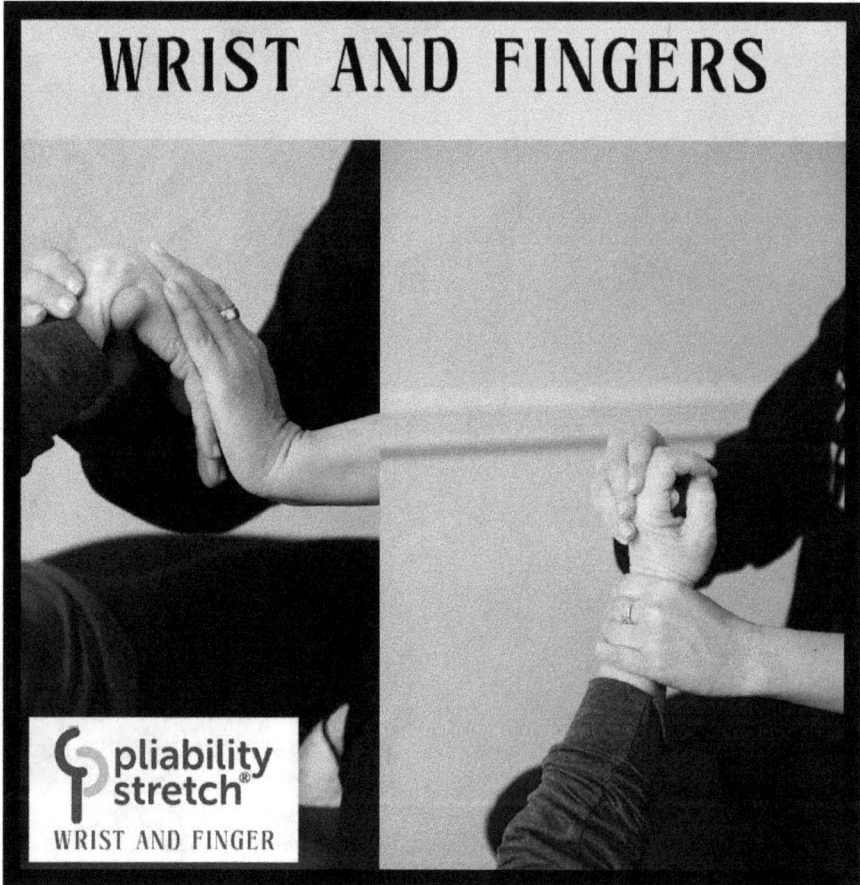

ANKLE STRETCH
Provide a simple calf stretch by pressing foot into flexion and extension.

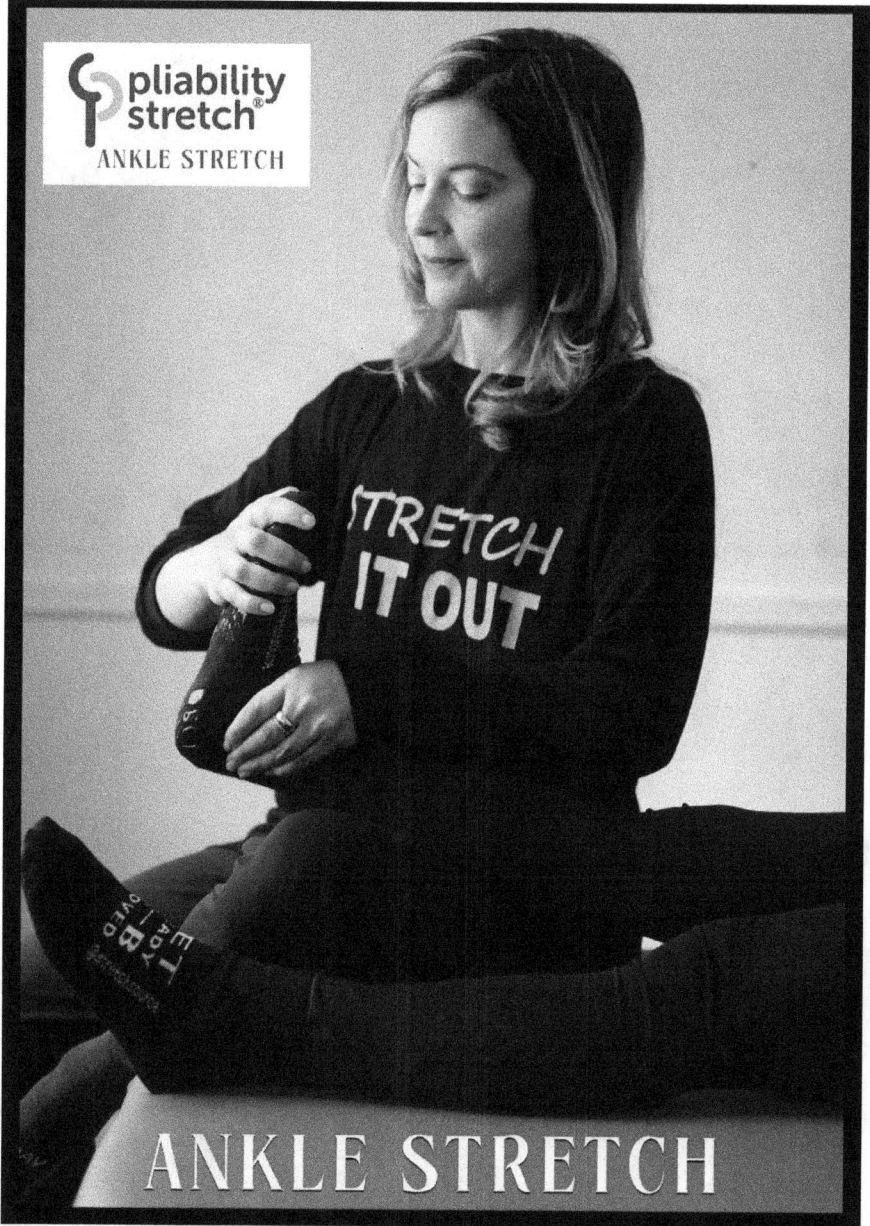

FINISH WITH FULL BODY STRETCH AND LEG SWINGS

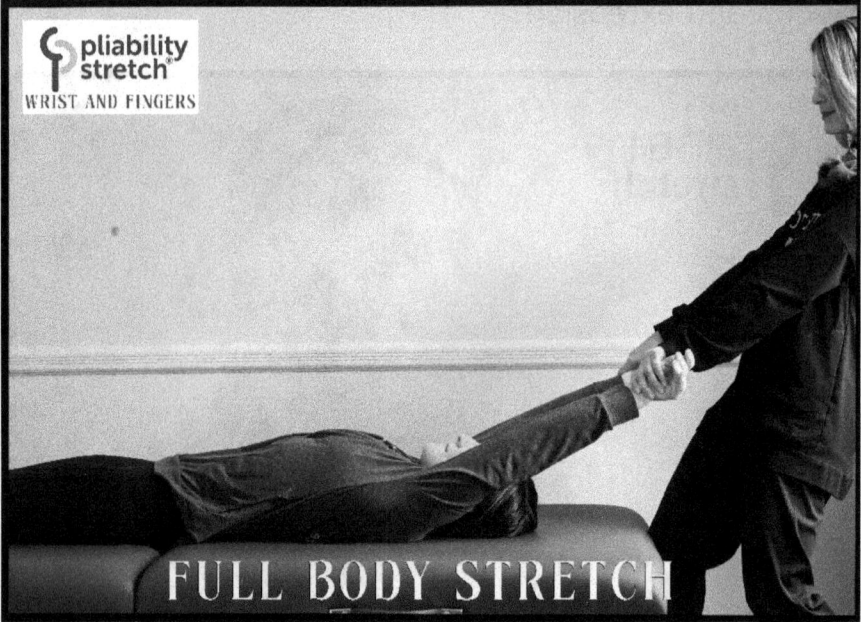

30 MINUTE SESSION

- WARM-UP (5 MINUTES)
- SERIES 1 (10 MINUTES)
- NO SERIES 2
- SERIES 3 (10 MINUTES)
- SERIES 4 (5 MINUTES)

60 MINUTE SESSION

- WARM-UP (10 MINUTES)
- SERIES 1 (15 MINUTES)
- SERIES 2 (10 MINUTES)
- SERIES 3 (15 MINUTES)
- SERIES 4 (10 MINUTES)

About the Author:

Mara Kimowitz, the creative mind and driving force behind Pliability Stretch® and Stretch Source®, is a trailblazer in the wellness and fitness industry. With a vision deeply rooted in enhancing individuals' well-being and flexibility, Mara pioneered these ventures to offer tailored stretch therapies and wellness solutions.

Drawing from a blend of expertise in dance, fitness, entrepreneurship, and holistic health, Mara has crafted unique approaches to wellness. Her dedication to providing effective stretch therapies and fostering a culture of wellness has positioned StretchSource® as go-to destinations for those seeking holistic rejuvenation.

Mara's relentless pursuit of innovation, coupled with her genuine passion for helping others achieve their health goals, sets her apart in the industry. Through her leadership and commitment, she continues to positively impact the lives of many, guiding them on their journey to optimal health and vitality.

Www.StretchSource.com
Www.pliabilitystretch.com

pliability
stretch®

UNLIMITED ACCESS TO DATABASE OF INSTRUCTIONAL VIDEOS

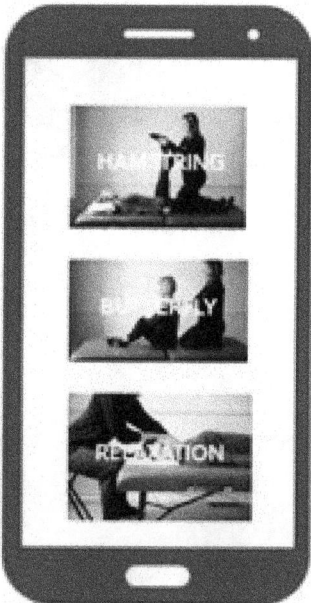

GET 14 DAYS FREE!